# Dog Training Basics

The Beginner's Guide to Raising the Perfect Dog with Positive Dog Training. Includes Puppy Training, Crate Training and Potty Training for Puppy

*Brandon White*

**Legal & Disclaimer**

whether directly or indirectly, of any advice or information presented, whether for breach of contract, tort, negligence, personal injury, criminal intent, or under any other cause of action.

You agree to accept all risks of using the information presented inside this book.

You agree that by continuing to read this book, where appropriate and/or necessary, you shall consult a professional (including but not limited to your doctor, attorney, or financial advisor or such other advisor as needed) before using any of the suggested remedies, techniques, or information in this book.

# Table of Contents

# Introduction

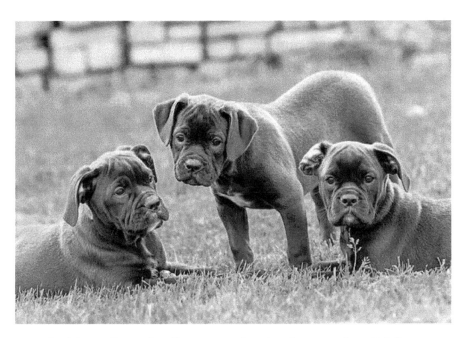

In primitive tribes, the first tamed animal was a dog. Wolves sought to stay close to people, counting on a share when hunting a large beast. These ancestors of dogs, as if themselves, came to man. Men very quickly realized that a tamed wolf has one very valuable quality - he can be a good assistant in hunting. The dog has done a great service to man, since the beginning of our union.

Dog breeding is currently gaining importance in various sectors of the economy. Dogs participate in the protection of objects, including the state border, and provide invaluable assistance to police officers. In the Far North, they are used as a vehicle.

Shepherd dogs protect flocks of sheep from the attack of predators, facilitate the work of shepherds during the hauls, and look after grazing animals. Dogs perform tasks of geologists, divers, signalmen, help disabled people, orderlies, rescuers, and many other ordinary and unusual assignments. They serve in the circus and participate in scientific expeditions. For example, experimental studies of academician, I.P. Pavlov, in the field of higher nervous activity were conducted on dogs. The effect of many drugs is studied and tested on them. Almost all methods that are currently used in the transplantation of organs and tissues in humans have been preliminarily worked out on dogs. Thousands of dogs have given their lives in the name of science. The dog even took an active part in space exploration.

Under the influence of centuries-old selection, the useful makings of dogs have been perfected in most modern breeds. These dog breeds are divided into three main groups - service, hunting, and indoor decorative dogs.

- Service dogs - German (East European), Caucasian, Central Asian, South Russian, Scottish shepherd dogs (collies), and others - are used for search, watch, guard, shepherding, and other services.

- Hunting dogs - West and East Siberian huskies, Karelian-Finnish huskies, and greyhounds are used for commercial and sport hunting.
- Room-decorative - poodles, lapdogs, and spitz are contained in apartments.

Whatever your dog breed, at least we all agree on one thing: they are ever faithful companions and are truly man's best friend.

To get the most out of your dog, however, it needs to be trained and "civilized." In this book is all you need to know to get the most out of your relationship with your loyal pet.

# Chapter 1

## Purchasing and Keeping a Dog. Puppy Selection

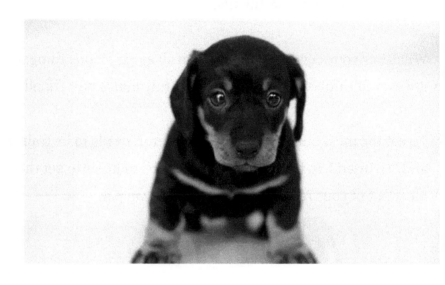

The acquisition of a dog is not simply a whim or a tribute to fashion. It is necessary to proceed, first of all, from one's professional interests and needs, psychological, and social opportunities. This requires a thorough assessment.

By acquiring a dog, a person assumes great moral responsibility. You need to be prepared for the fact that you have to spend a lot of time walking, grooming and feeding the dog, bear the material costs of veterinary care and various cosmetic procedures.

If you decide to buy a dog, do not purchase an adult animal. An adult dog may have physical disabilities, uncontrollable habits, and vices. A puppy, with proper upbringing and training, can become a physically developed, intelligent, well-trained dog devoted to its owner.

You should also not buy a dog in the market or from random people. A purebred puppy with an excellent pedigree, with good makings, healthy, and properly grown can be purchased at a registered dog breeding club. On such a puppy, over time, you will receive a document certifying its breed and origin.

If your family has middle-aged children and the puppy is designed for them, it is better to purchase a medium-sized dog, which can become a partner in games for the child, a companion during walks, and if necessary - a defender.

For those who need a gentle and affectionate dog, who, having laid his head on the owner's lap, will watch him adoringly for hours, one can recommend acquiring an Irish setter.

Terriers will become good moral support for people in a lonely house.

Of course, each owner seeks to acquire a full-fledged puppy and grow out of it a good, efficient, and thoroughbred dog. Therefore, he needs to know what it depends on.

The quality of the puppy depends on the features and abilities inherited from parents and immediate relatives (grandfathers, grandmothers, etc.), that is, on the genotype. The genotype is the hereditary constitution of an organism, the totality of its makings transmitted through chromosomes. By inheritance from the parents and immediate family, the puppy has transferred all the characteristic signs of the breed to which it belongs, as well as the features of the constitution, the exterior (appearance), and interior (growth, physique, behavior, training ability, etc.). In other words, the programmed basis for the growth and development of each puppy and the formation of an adult dog from it is its genotype. But much also depends on the conditions in which the puppy grows and develops on the quality of its maintenance, feeding, and upbringing. For example, the cowardice of a dog (fear of strong irritants) can be hereditary, transmitted from parents and immediate relatives (a weak type of higher nervous activity).

Limb defects expressed in varying degrees of weakness, lameness, improper posture (clubfoot, etc.) can arise from inherited defects (dysplasia of the hip joints) and rickets arising from malnutrition (deficiency in the daily diet vitamins D, A, calcium, phosphorus, etc.).

Depending on the genotype and the conditions of growth, development, and upbringing of the puppy, its phenotype develops. A phenotype is a set of all the signs and properties of an organism that are formed under the influence of hereditary factors and environmental conditions.

The phenotype of the puppy (constitution, exterior, behavioral features) that you have chosen will be formed depending on the genotype, hereditary inclinations received from parents and other close relatives, as well as under the influence of the external environment (keeping, feeding, raising) to which the significant degree is up to you. Therefore, it is necessary that the puppy, if possible, has high-breed parents, able to inherit pedigree, and has working qualities. It is necessary to create good conditions for him to be healthy, feed well, and be "educated." Only then will the high hereditary inclinations of the puppy be able to fully develop.

The puppy is exposed to the influence of the environment already in the prenatal period of its development which depends on the conditions of keeping and feeding the mother. The quality of a newly born puppy depends both on the makings transferred to him and on the conditions in which his mother was in the period of puppyhood.

When choosing a puppy, it is recommended to carefully examine him in order to find out if his breed is relevant, whether there are significant defects, physical development and activity for his age, as well as check the pedigree cards of parents, take an interest in the ratings that they received at exhibitions, competitions, if possible, establish their tribal class. It is recommended to find out the conditions of keeping and feeding the puppy's mother during puppyhood and feeding.

When choosing a puppy, you need to give preference to larger, well-fed, energetic puppies who are the first to get to the feeder and eat the food well.

It is recommended to take a puppy for growing no earlier than a month old, preferably at the age of 40–45 days. It is advisable to acquire a puppy at the end of spring and in the summer when the conditions for raising it are most favorable (heat, sun, lots of vegetables and herbs for vitamin top dressing, good conditions for walking, etc.).

When choosing a puppy, you could invite an experienced dog breeder, preferably a specialist in a service dog club who knows breeding dogs.

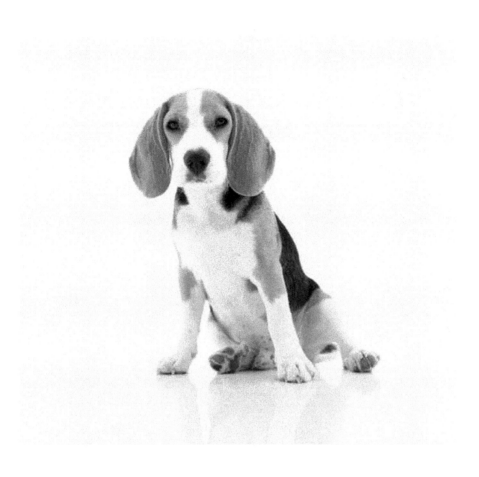

# Chapter 2

## How to Wean a Dog from Nibbling Home Things

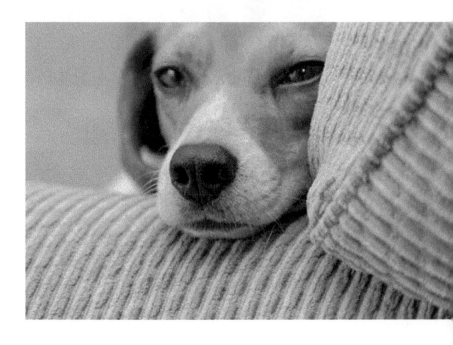

Once you have a puppy, take care of his upbringing. Usually, young dogs, out of curiosity, try to "taste" everything in a row, and if they are not weaned in a timely manner, then soon they will gnaw everything that is possible in your house. Thus, they not only satisfy their curiosity by studying objects but also escape from boredom.

If each time you only punish the dog, then you will not achieve a positive effect. The fact is that in an animal, the desire to gnaw and chew something is laid on an instinctive level. Punishment is perceived by him not as a prohibition to nibble at all, but as a prohibition to nibble while the owner is nearby. As soon as you leave the house, the dog again takes on his own. As a result, you get angry at don't understand "these stupid animals," instead of understanding dog instincts yourself. Each time you return home, you punish the dog, and as a result, it begins to fear your appearance and rejoice at your departure. If you punish a dog for a specific object damaged by it, it will stop nibbling it and take on another one (say, instead of a sofa, a chair). Therefore, the only way out is to show the animal what can be eaten.

The owner must give the dog several items with which it will play. As soon as the animal understands which toys can be nibbled, it immediately ceases to pay attention to other objects. But until the dog has recognized its toys, do not leave it in the house for a long time unattended. If you leave, close the dog in a separate room next to her things. While you are at home, occasionally look at what the dog is doing. If they are playing with their toys, praise her. If you are interested in something else, do not scold, but try to pay attention to her toy. When this is possible, be sure to praise the dog again. Thus, a conditioned reflex will form in the animal: the toy is praise, and the dog will stop biting your furniture.

As toys, it is advisable to use things that are difficult to chew, and impossible to swallow. The best materials are rawhide or hard rubber. It can be a ball, special artificial bone, and much more. Never use your old shoes or clothes as a toy, as the dog, playing with the old boot, will enthusiastically take on the new one.

If you leave the puppy alone unattended, give him a toy with a pleasantly smelling filling (but so that it is difficult to get it). The puppy will be so busy with the contents of the toy that, in your absence, will not pay attention to other objects in the house.

After the dog gets used to his toys, gets used to being alone, he can be safely left alone at home, not being afraid that he will start to howl or bite the furniture set.

# Chapter 3

## Dog Training Methods. Skills Development

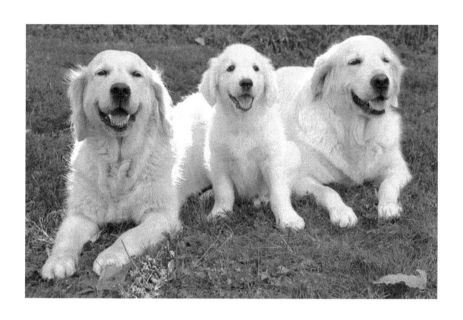

The first method is mechanical training. To obtain the desired unconditioned reflex, the trainer uses a mechanical stimulus (coercion). To make the dog sit down, you can accompany the "Sit!" command with strong hand pressure on the dog's hind. Showing a protective reflex, the dog will sit down. A repetition of this technique will develop a conditioned reflex in the animal, and the dog will sit down on the order of the trainer.

The mechanical stimuli used in dog training include pressing with a hand on various parts of the body, forcibly giving the body the desired position, jerking with a leash, jerking with the collar, or a slight blow with a whip.

The second method is palatable training. Food is used as an unconditioned irritant. The landing reflex is caused by raising a piece of meat above the dog's head. If such an effect is combined with the "Sit!" command and is accompanied by a treat, then a conditioned reflex will also form on the basis of the food unconditioned reflex. In the future, she will sit down only on the orders of the trainer.

The actions that the dog learns to perform in the process of training according to the signals of the trainer are more complicated than ordinary conditioned reflexes (for example, the conditioned reflex of salivation). Special studies have shown that these actions are complex motor reactions of the dog, consisting of a system of reflexes. Such complex actions of a dog are called skill. Skill is an individually acquired combination of unconditioned and conditioned reflexes.

When developing skills, the most appropriate is the contrast method of training, which consists of combining mechanical and taste-promoting methods. When practicing the skill, it is necessary, in addition to the unconditioned stimulus (food or mechanical), to use another stimulus. An unconditioned stimulus has the same meaning as in the development of a conditioned reflex, that is, it is a reinforcing stimulus. The effect of the second stimulus should cause a certain motor reaction. Thus, this stimulus will be prompting (pushing) to perform the desired action. This reaction is combined with the conditional signal of the trainer (command, gesture, etc.).

An analysis of skills formation shows that, in these cases, two conditioned reflexes are formed, which are closely related: firstly, a food reflex is established to a certain motor reaction of the dog, and this reaction, like a conditioned stimulus, begins to cause a food reflex (the dog sits down for order to get food); secondly, a conditional motor reaction (skill) is formed to perform this action on a signal. The irritating stimulus, originally used to induce a motor reaction, becomes redundant as soon as the dog begins to show this action on the command of the trainer.

For example, in order to train a dog to sit on the "Sit!" command based on the contrast method of training, you must first use two stimuli (mechanical and food).

A mechanical stimulus (pressing a hand on the hind) causes a landing (a defensive-defensive reflex in a passive form) and a food stimulus is the main unconditioned stimulus that reinforces the action by using a food unconditioned reflex. The "Sit!" command should be combined with the effects of both stimuli. It either precedes their action or is supplied simultaneously with the use of a mechanical stimulus. After the landing skill is formed on the "Sit!" command, the mechanical stimulus gradually loses its significance and the performed action should be supported only by a food irritant. A conditioned reflex forms on the "Sit!" command.

When using the method of mechanical training, the contrast value is also preserved. Here, the contrast is two different positions of the dog. One situation is associated with the action of a mechanical pain stimulus (a blow with a whip on the hind, pressure on the sacrum with a hand, a jerk with a leash). Another (the position of the completed landing) relieves the dog from the effects of a pain stimulus. Here, to reinforce a certain position of the dog, the main thing is the absence of negative, painful, irritation. This example shows well how ductile the higher nervous activity of the dog is (adaptation to environmental influences). Each trainer should remember that when using mechanical (especially pain) stimuli, reinforcement is not the action of the stimulus itself, but the disposal of it.

A distinctive feature of the skill is that the animal takes a more active part in the manifestation of this action: doing this movement on its own if it is a means of satisfying a vital need (finding food, stalking, and tracking down prey) or avoiding an action that could be dangerous to the body. Many skills, which are developed on the basis of the prevailing reactions and lead to the satisfaction of the dog's vital needs, appear much faster and become more durable than conditioned reflexes in laboratory experiments.

Remember though, a yard dog that was once beaten with a stick will always avoid a person with a stick in his hand.

As a stimulating (pushing) irritant when training dogs, you can use an already trained dog. In order to develop faster action in young dogs, a lesson can be done in the presence of an already trained adult dog. A young dog that needs to be trained to overcome obstacles is recommended to be brought to the site where it is trained with a well-trained dog. Her jump over an obstacle will serve as a stimulating (pushing) irritant for your dog. This method of training can be called imitative.

# Training Techniques

In each case, training according to one method or another is carried out using techniques. Each training session is divided into the following stages.

The first stage is the education of the initial action (the main conditioned reflex) on a specific conditioned stimulus (sound command, gesture, etc.). At this stage, the trainer must solve two problems: induce the dog to perform the desired action and work out the initial conditional connection to the action.

The first stage is characterized by two features. First, a generalization of conditioned stimuli may occur in a dog. The dog "still does not know how" to clearly distinguish and may exhibit erroneous actions, for example, lying down on the "Sit!" Command, etc. The trainer should "slow down" the dog's erroneous actions and secure only correctly performed actions with the goodies.

Secondly, at this stage, a strong connection to the action has not yet been established; the trainer cannot yet overcome the influence of distracting stimuli. Therefore, when educating the initial actions, classes should be conducted in an environment with the least amount of distracting stimuli.

The second stage is the complication of the initially developed action of the conditioned reflex to the skill. At the same time, actions complicating the initial conditioned reflex are added to the initial action brought up in the dog. For example, when a dog approaches the trainer by the command "Come!," such a complication is to fix its certain position at the trainer's left foot and establish a conditioned reflex on the gesture, endurance in various positions, etc.

In the second stage of training, environmental conditions should not be complicated. This provides quick and easy development of desired skills. It is necessary to ensure that the dog clearly distinguishes (differentiates) the applied commands, and timely "slow down" its erroneous actions. To do this, such actions are not reinforced by delicacy, but correctly performed - necessarily reinforced by encouragement.

The third stage is the consolidation of the practiced complex action (skill) in various environmental conditions. As soon as the dog is accustomed to clearly and without fail to perform all actions and the environment in which the classes are held, it is necessary to complicate, as often as possible, to change the location of the classes so that the new situation is necessarily associated with the presence of extraneous irritants (various sounds, the presence of people, animals, etc.). At first, in such conditions, the orienting reflex will intensely manifest in the dog, but gradually it will begin to fade and the dog will get used to new irritants. In order to control the dog's behavior in complicated conditions, the trainer should gradually use stronger measures of influence (increase the strength of the applied mechanical stimuli). In this case, it is necessary to give commands with threatening intonation.

When the dog is distracted and refuses to perform a certain action, the trainer should try to take into account the appropriate method of influencing the dog in these conditions.

Receptions consist of various, but strictly defined influences.

Dog training techniques for performing complex actions are based on the fact that animals gradually learn complex actions. The whole process of working with a dog is to implement a number of techniques. Moreover, each subsequent trick can be used only if, with the help of previous tricks, the animal has developed skills on the basis of which a new result (a more complex skill) can be obtained.

When training guard dogs, it is necessary to develop maliciousness and distrust of people in them, to train them to work on a short leash, etc.

# Requirements for the Trainer

In the process of training, the main factor in organizing the behavior of the dog is the trainer. He not only affects the behavior of the dog but also seeks to complete actions that ensure its "official" use. The success of the work depends on the theoretical preparedness of the trainer and his practical experience. The trainer must correctly and quickly solve problems arising in the process of training, and remember the need for an individual approach to the dog. This is primarily due to a careful attitude to work, and attention, as you know, is the basis of observation, without which it is impossible to study the behavior of the animal. In order to develop observability, the trainer must keep a diary to note the results achieved and the characteristic features of the dog's behavior, as well as the mistakes made by the trainer himself.

The methods and techniques used in the training process should be applied differently in each case. Without this, an individual approach to the dog is unthinkable.

In order to skillfully control the actions of the dog, the trainer must be strictly consistent in work. When starting to develop one or another skill in a dog, it is necessary to outline which method and technique should be used and to think through the sequence of your actions well. Having started training the dog, it is necessary to persistently carry out the tasks. Various changes and additions arising in the process of training should be strictly justified. As much as possible, the training process must be built taking into account existing methodological principles.

When training, various difficulties often arise. The reasons that cause them may depend on the behavior of the dog or the unforeseen environmental effects. In order to quickly make the right decision, the trainer must know the theoretical foundations and practical techniques for working with the dog and skillfully apply them.

During practical training, the trainer should strive to maintain the dog's "interest" in the work. For this, it is necessary to take into account the general condition of the dog (health, the degree of its excitability, the presence of estrus, etc.), not to overwork it and diversify the methods of training. Of great importance are the skillful use and combination of coercion, encouragement, and prohibition. Each trainer should have endurance, resourcefulness, courage, and strictly observe the sequence of his actions. The success of training depends largely on the love for animals. Therefore, the best option is when the owner is training the dog.

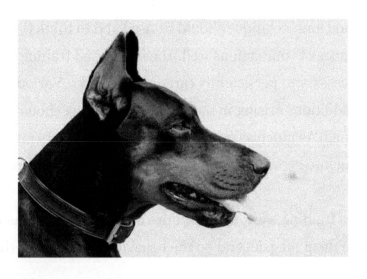

# Chapter 4

## Training Rules

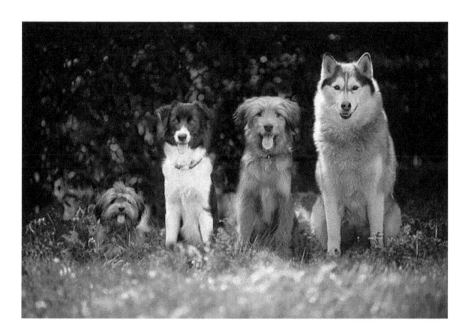

The trainer must strictly adhere to the following rules:

1.  Starting training, you need to carefully study the characteristics of the dog's behavior (a type of higher nervous activity, the predominant reaction), accustom the animal to itself (make it relaxed, sort of), and only after that, you can start to work.

2.  At each lesson, it is necessary to set a specific task and seek to achieve it.

3. Strictly observe the basic rule for the development of a conditioned reflex to apply a conditioned stimulus (command, gesture) somewhat earlier than an unconditioned, in extreme cases, simultaneously.

4. Do not change the commands, but use the appropriate intonation and carefully monitor the correctness and clarity of the commands and gestures.

5. Not to be nervous to avoid rudeness and excessive affection, to be demanding and persistent, and not forgetting to encourage every correct action of the dog.

6. Training should be carried out according to the principle: "from simple to complex."

7. Not to tire the dog with the uniformity of exercises, to diversify the activities, and try to maintain the dog's interest in performing various actions.

8. Closely monitor the physical condition of the animal.

## Weather Conditions and their Impact on Working with a Dog

Dog training takes place in various weather conditions. Some of them make it easier, others make it difficult to work with the dog. Training should always begin in light conditions, gradually complicating them and achieving trouble-free operation.

Under environmental conditions that facilitate or complicate the work with a dog, one should understand the time of day, temperature, wind speed, soil condition, and the nature of the terrain.

It is recommended to work with a dog in the early morning. At this time, the animal feels well after a night's rest and the environment is very favorable (few outsiders, animals, etc.). In the morning hours (especially in summer), the air is cool and heat exhausts the dog. Accustoming the animal to work in hot weather should be gradual. However, training during daylight hours provides the best control by the trainer as there is maximum visibility. It should be borne in mind that in the dark, the alertness and protective reflexes of the dog are better manifested, therefore, guard and watchdogs should be trained at dusk and at night.

High or low air temperature strongly affects the dog's body, and heat acts more negatively than cold (in the absence of drafts and wind). Positive results of training can be achieved by gradually accustoming the dog to work at high or low temperatures. Go to work at higher or lower temperatures gradually. Generally, dogs with adequate nutrition can easily tolerate low temperatures.

To take into account the influence of the wind, it is necessary to distinguish between its direction (passing, oncoming, lateral, angular) and strength (in points). To work with the dog, the headwind of small force is most favorable. It facilitates the work of guard and watchdogs. The direction and strength of the wind are extremely important for the dog to track. The nature of the soil cover is especially important for the training and work of search dogs. It is necessary to distinguish between favorable and unfavorable soils. Favorable soils include slightly wet, slightly loosened, meadow, forest, clay, peat and snow cover, while unfavorable includes rocky, dry, sandy, and swampy (flooded with water).

The nature of the terrain is determined by the topography, vegetation, and population. On flat terrain, the dog is easier to work with; heavily rugged terrain makes it difficult to act. The presence of vegetation may, in some cases, be a favorable factor and in others, a negative one. For example, a well-developed, low grass cover facilitates trail work. A small but sparse shrub develops a dog's search activity in the forest where air movement is limited. However, too thick and tall grass, as well as a dense shrub, impede the dog's movement, the animal gets tired faster. In addition, plants with a strong stupefying smell (for example, rosemary), which negatively affect the higher nervous activity of the animal, are often found in the grass.

Strongly changing terrain contributes to the development of the dog, but it quickly tires. Therefore, in the initial training, dogs must be taught on level ground. In settlements, the work of dogs is complicated. This is due to a large number of distracting irritants. Therefore, the dog must be gradually accustomed to working in such conditions on the principle of "from simple to complex."

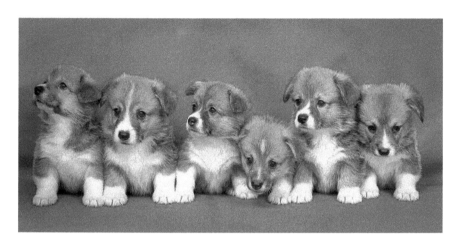

## Possible Trainer Errors

In the process of training, the trainer may allow various erroneous actions in relation to the dog. The trainer's mistakes complicate the training and reduce its quality; in the future, they can become an obstacle to the use of a dog.

The causes of possible errors may be poor theoretical training of the trainer, insufficient practical experience, and lack of analysis of the training process.

Most often, trainers make the following mistakes.

1. Underestimate or overestimate the behavior of dogs. This is due to the subjective approach to the animal, in addition, the qualitative difference between the higher nervous activity of a person and a dog is ignored. The trainer "humanizes" the dog. He ascribes to her the ability to consciously relate to his actions, etc. Such a trainer, in addition to the prescribed commands, begins to persuade the dog to perform one or another action, even threatens her.

   Such actions make it difficult to develop conditioned reflexes to the corresponding command, as the sounds are mixed with other sounds (words). You should know, with extraneous sound stimuli, the dog is distracted (tentative reaction), which inhibits the execution of various commands.

   The trainer, attributing to the dog the ability to consciously understand the meaning of the words of the command, begins to misuse the commands as certain conditioned stimuli. For example, prompting the dog to take the ball item by the "Ball!" Command, he, taking this item from the dog's mouth, uses more than one "Give!" Command, but says: "Give the ball!." Essentially, there is a violation of the basic principle of developing a conditioned reflex. The dog has a conditioned reflex of grasping the subject on the "Ball!"

command. This command means for the dog the need to keep a round item in its mouth. The command "Give!" is a conditional irritant for the dog to give the subject to the trainer. Therefore, the simultaneous use of the commands "Give!" And "Give the ball!" will be perceived as the simultaneous execution of two mutually exclusive actions "give" and "take." Such an incorrect combination of the two named actions makes it difficult to develop the necessary skill in a dog and a breakdown of nervous activity can occur.

2. Another error is possible. Suppose that while walking without a leash, the dog was distracted by an extraneous stimulus (cat, bird, other dogs, etc.) and did not approach the trainer by the command "Come," but only after several repeated commands. If you punish the dog (at the time of approaching the trainer), the basic principle of developing a conditioned reflex to the "Come!" command will be violated, which is based on the food reflex and getting treats when approaching the trainer. Punishment of the dog when approaching the trainer will cause her a defensive reflex, and in the future, the animal will be afraid to approach him. In addition, the dog will be afraid of a leash in the hands of a trainer. It will also slow down her approach to him.

It must be remembered that punishing a dog (as a person understands it) is completely unacceptable. In training, it is not a punishment that is used, but "prohibition."

Underestimating the dog's "abilities" (higher nervous activity) is usually the result of ignorance of the type of higher nervous activity and the prevailing reactions of the animal. Because of this, the individual approach to the dog during training is ignored, the greatest suitability of the dog for a certain type of service is not taken into account; the template approach to animals is used in the training process. The same training methods are unacceptable for dogs of various types of higher nervous activity (excitable, calm, spiteful, cowardly, with a predominance of food reaction and without it). Without an individual approach to animals in the process of training, it is difficult to achieve an effect on work, you can spoil a dog.

The main condition for the development of a conditioned reflex is a consistent combination of conditioned and unconditioned stimuli. In this case, the conditioned stimulus (command) must precede the unconditioned stimulus or appear simultaneously with it.

However, inexperienced trainers often break this rule. They do not take into account the fact that in the case when the conditioned stimulus is applied after the unconditioned, the development of the conditioned reflex is difficult. A gross error of the trainer is the abuse of one or another action in the process of training. Having not achieved a strongly conditioned reflex to the action, the trainer begins to repeat it many times, without simultaneously using the necessary unconditional "reinforcement." He thinks that the dog will perform the required action. In fact, such repeated use of the command without an unconditional irritant will cause her to gradually weaken (fade) the conditioned reflex to the action and lead to the fact that she does not develop faultlessness and accuracy of the skill.

Very often, trainers underestimate the importance of intonation and pronounce commands in the same intonation. As a result, the trainer loses the ability to use intonation as a very important auxiliary stimulus that enhances the action of the action.

To avoid this error, you should initially give a command with the usual (ordered) intonation. When the dog does not perform the action, the command with threatening intonation should be repeated; if the command is still not executed, you need to repeat it again with threatening intonation and reinforce it with an unconditional mechanical stimulus (pressing, snatch leash, strict collar tug, slight whip or blow).

However, you cannot often abuse the threatening intonation - this will lead to the fact that the dog will cease to respond t it. In the process of training, one should often force a dog with strong mechanical and painful stimuli (especially a strict collar tug and whip). It is not recommended to show an overly affectionate and undemanding attitude towards the dog: the animal ceases to obey the trainer.

Using treats for encouragement, one should not stroke the dog and exclaim "Good!" with gentle intonation. This will no allow to gradually limit the giving of goodies and to widely use other rewards. Abuse of delicacy leads to the fact that the dog, waiting for it, "is distracted by the trainer" and accustomed to execute commands only with food reinforcement.

3. The harshest mistake of the trainer is unnecessary haste, which entails fuzzy training and insufficient reinforcement c skills. As a result, persistent conditioned reflexes to the command are not developed, so the trainer cannot control the dog's behavior, especially in difficult conditions and successfully carry out training.

It is recommended to avoid repeating fixed skills of the same sequence. This contributes to the formation of a strong conditioned reflex connection to a certain system of actions (stereotype), and the dog ceases to obey the trainer. If, for example, you let a dog in the same sequence to overcome obstacles, she will "remember" this sequence and begin to overcome obstacles one after another only at the first command, not stopping before each obstacle.

## Neuroses and Unwanted Connections

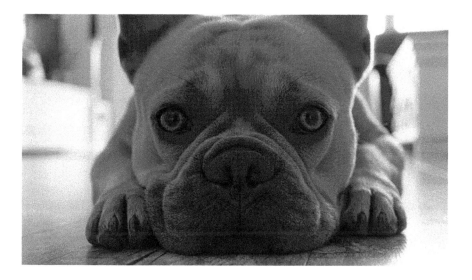

As a result of the erroneous actions of the trainer and his incorrect approach to the dog, the higher nervous activity of the animal may be disturbed. In the process of training, these disorders are most often manifested in dogs in the form of neuroses and unwanted connections.

Neurosis is a functional violation of nervous activity without visible damage to the nervous system. The most common cause of neurosis in dogs is a breakdown of nervous activity - a pathological violation of the processes of excitation and inhibition in the cerebral cortex.

Disruption of a dog's nervous activity can occur. In different dogs, neurosis is characterized by various signs of behavior. Some animals in a state of neurosis show increased excitement and "irritability" (they easily go into an aggressive state even in relation to a trainer, show poor differentiation). Others have a depressed state. They become fearful and distrustful. An increased voice or a sharp cry of a trainer causes a prolonged inhibitory state in such animals.

Some dogs exhibit a pronounced tendency to stiffness and drowsiness, they become less susceptible to commands and other effects of the trainer.

Disruption of nervous activity and subsequent neurosis can also occur as a result of overstrain of nervous processes of excitation and inhibition. Overexertion of the processes of excitation most often occurs when the dog's nervous system is exposed to super strong stimuli (for example, shots and explosions), if the animal is not previously accustomed to them; with abuse of coercion (the use of strong pain stimuli without regard to the type of higher nervous activity).

In the case of neurosis in the dog's behavior, actions incomprehensible to the trainer can sometimes occur. She can, for example, show cowardice in relation to people dressed in a certain suit; without being afraid of men, can be afraid of women or children, etc. or begin to attack or show cowardice only in the presence of a dog of a certain breed, etc. The reason for these incomprehensible phenomena in the behavior of dogs suffering from neurosis was explained by the studies of academician Pavlov. It turns out that the external manifestation of neurosis is often associated with "strong impressions" (nervous injuries) experienced by the dog long before the breakdown of nervous activity. It happens, for example, that in a state of neurosis, an adult dog begins to be afraid of puppies. This happens, apparently, because, in the past, she was bitten by a small dog.

The occurrence of neurosis directly depends on the type of higher nervous activity of the animal. Most often, persistent neurosis occurs in dogs of extreme types - excitable and weak. Balanced type dogs are more resistant to neurosis.

To cure a neurosis, you can temporarily stop training with a dog, transfer it to another trainer (other conditions of employment), and use medicines (bromine).

Unlike neurosis, an unwanted connection cannot be considered as a pathological condition of the nervous system. An unwanted connection is a conditioned reflex that a dog has experienced against the trainer's desire as a result of his mistakes. This not only complicates the training but also creates great obstacles to the "official" use of dogs.

Consider the causes of the most common unwanted relationships in dogs. When training in the general course, it is necessary to accustom the dog to the precise execution of action by command and gesture separately. Gestures are most often taught based on previously assigned sound commands. Combining commands with gestures is permissible only at the beginning of training. In the future, you should use commands and gestures separately. Without taking this into account, many novice trainers combine a gesture with an action for a long time. In this case, the dog forms an undesirable connection to perform actions only on a complex stimulus (command + gesture).

With the development of viciousness in dogs, it is necessary to ensure that the assistants do not always work in a training gown. Otherwise, the dog develops an unwanted connection, and it will attack or listen to a person in only such clothes.

If practical training also takes place in the same environment for a long time, the dog may have an undesirable relationship. As a result of this, once in a new place, she will refuse to fulfill the requirements of the trainer.

The main methods to combat the occurrence of unwanted relationships:

1. A thorough analysis of all the tricks and effects of the trainer used during training;
2. A change in the environment in which an unwanted connection arose, and the elimination of the stimuli that caused its appearance;
3. The temporary cessation of practical training in certain ways until the conditioned reflex to an undesirable connection fades.

# Chapter 5
## What You Need to Have in Mind!

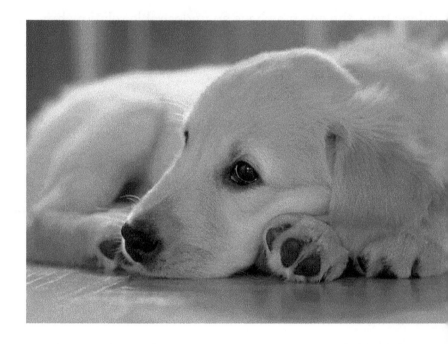

Many dogs experience bouts of panic fear of loneliness. Such attacks occur in those animals that are very strongly attached to their master, who from childhood has been accustomed to being close to him all the time and needs constant attention. This is quite common in adopted dogs. The fear of loneliness in a dog arises in puppyhood. The reason may be a move to a new home or training location or frequent care of the owner for a long time

Symptoms of a panic state are as follows. The dog's breathing quickens and the heart rate and heartbeat increases. Often, there are attacks of suffocation, excessive salivation, involuntary discharge of feces and urine, and heavy sweating. Vomiting is sometimes possible.

Often, the animal seeks to prevent the owner from leaving with an aggressive imitation of attack and a loud bark. If the owner has nevertheless left, the dog begins to howl loudly. Therefore, when you hear the howling of a neighboring dog, then most likely it suffers from a fear of loneliness and awaits the arrival of its beloved owner. All these symptoms begin to appear within 20-30 minutes after the animal is left alone.

When the owner comes, the dog greets him with a loud bark, jumps and runs around him, and follows him on his heels from room to room.

In order to cure the dog of bouts of panic and fear of loneliness, you need a whole complex of retraining of the animal. First of all, the dog needs to be reassured with antidepressants and tranquilizers. After the animal calmed down, you can begin retraining.

First of all, start by gradually accustoming the dog to care. To do this, dress, take a bag, and go out (walk the dog) for 5-10 minutes. In such a short time, the animal is unlikely to have fear. With each departure, increase its duration by 5-10 minutes until the dog gets used to your long absences.

Leave the animal in those places at home where it feels more or less safe and calm. Put his favorite toys there before leaving. You can also turn on soft melodious music. Before leaving, try not to play with the dog, so as not to excite it in vain.

When you go to bed, close the animal's access to your bedroom. It is advisable that the dog sleeps in its place. It will also help her get used to your absences.

## Phobias

In addition to fear of loneliness, many dogs often have a fear of phenomena incomprehensible to them. For example, the animal is afraid of lightning strikes, thunderstorms, fire, etc. In these situations, it is best to give the dog antidepressants and tranquilizers as calming agents. In addition, try to gradually accustom the dog to noise, and each time, praise her for her courage.

# How to Distinguish an Aggressive Dog

Among the most aggressive breeds of dogs are pit bulls, Caucasian, Central Asian, German shepherd dogs, Rottweilers as well as dogs crossed with these breeds. Usually, groomed dogs that have not been walked for a long time tend to be aggressive. It is also similar for dogs in a pack and without a leash. Strange as it may seem, stray dogs attack much less frequently (the exception is sick with rabies or animals forced to defend themselves). Sometimes, familiar dogs bite. Most often, animals bite animals. Usually, during games with dogs, children inattentively hurt them (pull their tail, step on their paws, etc.), and the animal instinctively begins to defend itself.

It must be remembered that when a dog is about to attack, it exposes incisors and fangs. Such a grin has nothing to do with a "smile," so try not to annoy the animal. It is best to move a safe distance from it.

Very often, dogs attack with a sense of fear (believing that the subject of the attack is fraught with danger). In such cases, the animal slightly arches its back, tightens its tail, slightly snaps its teeth, exposes its fangs and incisors, and presses its ears to the head. Usually, a dog only simulates an attack (forepaws are widely spaced, muzzle is slightly lowered, head is located at back level). But remember that even in imitation, she is always ready to bite you. At the same time, the dog tries not to look into your eyes, and if it is not annoying, there will be no attack. The main thing is to not turn your back to the animal.

If the animal's ears are sticking up, its mouth is bared, wrinkles appear on the face (around the eyes and on the forehead), and the nose is extended, this means that the dog is not afraid of you and is ready to attack. The coat of an aggressively tuned dog is raised, the eyes turn red and become cloudy, the pupil expands, and the animal stares intently into your eyes. Pay attention to the tail of the dog. If it is raised up and moves energetically, the animal is confident in its victory and the probability of attack increases.

The dog's worst weapon is its jaw. First of all, try to protect yourself from the teeth of the animal. Claw scratches are not so dangerous and will heal quickly. But with its teeth, a dog can no only bite through soft tissues but can also crush your bone.

## How to avoid a dog attack

Here are some basic tips for raising a dog that will help overcome its excessive aggressiveness.

From an early age, teach your dog obedience. She must know exactly what she is not allowed to do and know her responsibilities. If you bought a dog, not for hunting and not for guard purposes, try not to raise aggressiveness in it. If your dog belongs to breeds that are aggressive by nature, walk it only on a leash and in a muzzle. Walk it regularly, otherwise, the animal becomes embittered. In no case, do not set a dog on a person "as a joke" - the time will come and she will rush at someone seriously. Do not let your ward be in the pack - the animal can quickly run wild. If the dog's aggressiveness is pathological, it must be neutered.

In order not to anger the dog, follow simple rules. Do not touch the dog while sleeping or eating. Never take food or a toy from her. Do not separate the fighting dogs with your bare hands. Do not come close to the dog guarding its pups. Do not get close to a dog who is in his house or in the owner's car. Do not look directly into the eyes of an unfamiliar dog. Never run away from the attacked dog, it only provokes her to continue the attack. In case of an attack, stand still, do not move your hands, try to calmly talk with the dog. If you scream at her, trying to drive her away, this will further anger the animal.

If the dog still attacked you, lie down on the ground, pull your knees up to the chin, and try to protect your throat and head with your hands. And most importantly, keep children away from dogs. Follow the behavior of the animal during its games with children.

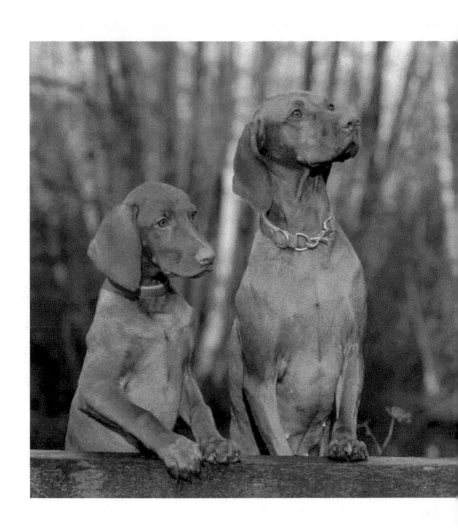

# Chapter 6
## Introduction to the General Training Course

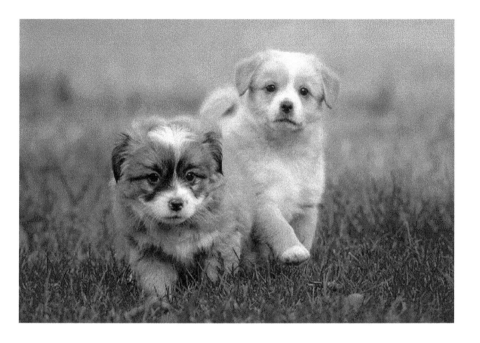

Raising a puppy means developing his skills and habits that are useful to the owner. This is the training of a puppy to perceive, in a timely manner, the stimuli of the external and internal environment and correctly respond to them in order to facilitate its daily maintenance and subsequent training. At the same time, during the upbringing, the puppy is inhibited and you thus eliminate unnecessary, bad habits. This achieves a puppy behavior that is convenient for the owner, members of his family, and those around him.

Under the initial training, which is sometimes called educational, understand the development of the puppy's conditioned reflexes and initial skills that allow using commands and gestures to control his behavior. Unlike adult dog training, the initial training of puppies does not aim to teach them to immediately, clearly, and without fail to execute commands in any environmental conditions, but only to respond to them correctly and to perform, even if not clear enough. The puppy is raised during the period of its cultivation and initial training, and these processes are closely intertwined.

The success of upbringing depends primarily on the conditions in which the puppy grows and develops. If these conditions are favorable (the puppy is kept in a bright, dry, fairly spacious and airy room, has a full daily diet, is provided with long walks and games every day), then it grows well and develops, and can be successfully brought up. And vice versa, if the puppy insufficiently grows up physically developed and pained, then the process of education will be less effective.

The success of upbringing largely depends on how well it is methodically built and implemented, which, in turn, is determined by the preparedness of the owner - the puppy's educator, his relevant knowledge, and experience.

The owner should know the basics of the psychophysiology of behavior and dog training. This will allow him to correctly and competently handle his pet and effectively act on him in order to develop useful skills and inhibit the bad skills and habits. We strongly recommend that you carefully read the appropriate training sections in this book before you have a puppy.

Obeying instincts, a newly born puppy, still deaf and blind, finds a mother's nipple, crawls towards her or other puppies to warm herself, and whines to attract her mother's attention.

From the age of 3 weeks, the puppy begins self-education (acquiring his own experience and developing appropriate skills). Collective games and walks under the supervision of the mother, as well as individual active movements around the apartment and in the yard under the supervision of the owner, are useful for its development.

The bitch encourages puppy games and interrupts them if the puppies start biting each other badly. During walks, she teaches the puppies, by her own example, to avoid dangerous pits, overcome low obstacles, and being aware of strangers and animals.

Building relationships with the puppy needs to be thoughtful, balanced, and reasonable. Cold, rude, and overly affectionate actions bring equal harm.

For the puppy to develop interest, activity, and courage during the game, he needs to periodically give in, imitating his victory. However, this should not be abused, as the puppy can believe that the owner is really afraid of him, that he is weaker. In no case should the owner allow the puppy to bite, even the weak ones. Relationships with the puppy need to be built in such a way that he clearly understands who is the owner whom he must protect, and whom to obey. The puppy should treat its owner as a leader.

If during the game the puppy tries to break the line of what is permitted by biting the owner, etc., he needs to be distracted from unwanted actions by switching to another occupation. If this does not succeed, it is necessary to take prohibitive measures, easily slapping his palm, or hitting him with a twig on the back. Otherwise, some dogs, especially aggressive breeds (Caucasian, Shepherd Dogs, etc.) will actually try to take the upper hand over the owner and begin to use their teeth, becoming uncontrollable "dictators" that are dangerous for family and others.

Initial training of the puppy and his upbringing are not intended to teach him to sit down, lie down, stand, etc. (he can do this thanks to natural inclinations), but are needed so that the puppy learns to perform such actions on the command of the owner.

The first lessons for puppies are given by their mother. The main task of the owner of the puppy is to continue its upbringing in order to prepare the 8 to a 10-month-old puppy for the successful development of the general training course, and in the future, one or another course of special training. The importance of education cannot be underestimated or ignored, as what is lost at this age cannot be caught up. If you do not educate your puppy, he will inevitably develop bad habits, many of which cannot be eradicated.

In puppies, especially at the age of 3-4 months, the body and nervous system are very susceptible to educational influence on the part of the owner. It is unreasonable to miss such an opportune moment since what could be achieved from the puppy will later require great efforts from the trainer or even become unattainable.

It is almost impossible to draw a clear line between raising a puppy and its initial training, however, these processes differ in their tasks and implementation methods. Especially sharply raising a puppy differs from training an adult dog.

The general thing for education and training is that they are aimed at developing a dog's skills and habits that are useful for a person and preventing unnecessary and harmful actions.

The difference between education and training is as follows. During the upbringing, the task is to develop common initial useful skills for a person that make the puppy obedient in everyday communication and are the basis for the subsequent initial training, and then, when the puppy grows up, they become the basis for successful general and special training. Thus, the goal of education is to develop initial obedience, the basic elements of discipline, which are far from perfect. Training makes it possible for puppies to develop clear, trouble-free skills not only in general obedience but also in a general and special training course, which will allow them to be used in one or other service (work).

It is necessary to take into account the fact that the behavior and development of a puppy are very different from an adult dog. H has not yet been sufficiently formed and strengthened; his life experience is not great. During classes, he quickly gets tired and reacts sharply to strong external stimuli. In addition, puppies are very different from each other depending on age. Therefore, the upbringing and initial training of each puppy should be carried out strictly individually, taking into account age characteristics.

All effects on puppies, especially up to 3-4 months of age, should be gentle. Mechanical effects can be used, but rarely and carefully, if you cannot do without them. More often, to develop the necessary skills, you should use a treat, games, or imitation of the actions of trained dogs. Significant blows in strength and pain, as well as overly loud prohibiting commands, will frighten the puppy and disrupt contact with the owner.

When executing commands periodically, at first more often, then less often, but in all cases, immediately exclaim "Good!" and give a treat. Increase the duration of the exercises and increase the requirements for the puppy to be gradual. In no case can you get trouble-free and clear action from him, like from an adult dog.

Overuse of activities with a puppy will lead to overwork, loss of ability to develop and improve the necessary skills, and disruption of higher nervous activity. If the puppy looks tired, classes should be stopped until the next day.

To prevent overwork, even if the puppy begins to lose interest in classes, you can resort to regular 5-minute breaks during which the puppy can run free.

# Methods and Techniques of Education and Initial Training

Raising a puppy and its initial training should be done from the first day after it has been taken away from the mother, and up to 8-10 months of age, when you should proceed to a systematic general course of training.

After the puppy has been taken away from his mother and separated from his peers, he needs constant communication with people. In the early days, he very painfully endures separation from relatives, since dogs belong to the number of animals living in packs in natural conditions. First, the puppy will be bored, asks for his friends by whining, and persistently avoids the space reserved for him. Despite this, the owner must continue to educate - do not pick up the puppy in his arms or do not let him into bed or on the sofa. If the puppy is very restless, you need to play with him, stroke him, calm him down, and allow him to lie down at the owner's feet.

The successful upbringing of a puppy is possible only if he has one owner who is engaged in cleaning and feeding, walking, and systematically training him. Family members for these purposes can be involved only if the owner is away or sick. You can't take care of raising a puppy in turn, because each person has his own ideas about the methods of education, and the puppy is not able to adapt to such a variety of approaches. An exception to this rule may be cases when the puppy is very "guilty" in the absence of the owner, which must be stopped immediately. Infrequent walking and feeding of the puppy by family members is allowed.

When choosing a site for classes, you should ensure that there is no debris or objects that could injure the puppy. If there is no special need, it is not necessary to force the puppy to sit down or lie down on the dirty ground.

It is a mistake to believe that raising a puppy is limited only to developing skills for him on the commands "Sit!," "Lie!," "Come!," and others because most of the useful skills are developed during walking, cleaning, and feeding. Walks are especially useful for this purpose, during which the puppy has the opportunity to meet various people, animals, and see vehicles which allows him to gradually get used to and calmly respond to such irritants, as well as learn to avoid dangers. If during a walk the puppy is frightened of something, he needs to be stroked and reassured. Try to distract him with a game and change the route, discreetly bring him to the object that frightened him to give him the opportunity to sniff it.

Each puppy should receive the necessary education. However, educational methods should be applied depending on the purpose for which it is grown. Puppies intended for search, protective, and guard services need to bring up a pronounced active-defensive reaction to strangers. It is impossible to allow that outsiders caress, feed him, or play with him. After 3–4 months of age, such puppies should be treated uninterestedly yet calmly, and in the future, with age, even with caution. Puppies should not show fear and anger. Do not bother them for a short time when they bark outsiders entering the apartment. However, you must not allow strangers to show pronounced threatening actions to the puppies, since repeated repetition of them in dogs may develop increased viciousness or severe cowardice. Cowardly dogs are generally not suitable for training.

If puppies are trained for purposes that do not require an active defensive reaction, they should be kind to people, so you should not prohibit petting such puppies by outsiders.

Dogs are born with their own individual characteristics. As a result, some puppies are easier to train and educate than others. Adult dogs also differ in their ability to train and work. However, even taking into account this pattern, one cannot blame a puppy for misconduct, since in the overwhelming majority of cases its owner is guilty, who devotes insufficient time to his education and feeding.

If a puppy eats stucco, food waste, or sewage at home or during a walk, you first need to find out if he receives enough minerals from the food, and if not, you need to increase the mineral feeding, paying attention not only to the number of minerals but also on their assortment. The puppy's body must receive sufficient calcium, phosphorus, trace elements, and other minerals.

If despite good nutrition the puppy continues to eat plaster, pick up food waste, and lick the ground, precautionary educational measures should be taken. On a walk along the chosen route, you need to layout pieces of meat, bone, etc., in advance, marking these places with sticks and branches invisible to the puppy. On a walk, you need to carefully monitor him and, as soon as he tries to grab the bone, you should immediately say the prohibiting command "No!" and make a sensitive jerk with a leash. Such actions need to be repeated 2-3 times.

Very often, puppies scratch and gnaw the plaster, furniture, wallpaper, if they are left alone for a long time. Therefore, you need to try not to leave them or give them in the absence of the owner. When trying to perform these actions, you should immediately pronounce the prohibiting command "No!" and try to distract the puppy with the game. If the puppy does not obey, he can be lightly hit with a twig on the back.

Most puppies like to jump on the owner, leaning on him with his front paws. To avoid this, when promoting, one should not raise the food too high so that the puppy does not bounce after it and does not rest its paws on the owner. If the habit has nevertheless appeared, it must be stopped by the forbidding command "No!," and if the puppy does not obey, you can simply hit him with a twig on the back.

It is not recommended to allow the puppy to lick the owner's face, as this is unhygienic. At the same time, the puppy should not be prohibited from periodically licking its hands, after which, they should be naturally washed with soap.

So that the puppy does not beg, when the owners eat, it needs to be fed beforehand, and every attempt to get closer to the table is immediately stopped by the "Place!" command. If the puppy does not respond to the command, it should be repeated and the puppy should be put in its place.

The puppy must correctly respond to meeting with strangers. In no case should he be allowed to perceive strangers he met on the street as friends or, even worse, as enemies or show fear. Puppies up to 2-3 months of age, as a rule, are friendly to strangers. Do not stop them from getting to know each other because, in this way, they gain life experience. At the same time you must not allow an outsider to caress the puppy or play with him. This will help the puppy develop a calm and disinterested attitude towards people.

Puppies that have reached 3 months of age have individual behavior. Most of the puppies do not show much interest to outsiders, much less joy, and become alert. Some puppies bark at intruders, which should be encouraged by stroking and exclaiming "Good!.." However, long barking should not be encouraged. If the puppy was frightened of incoming outsiders who make sudden movements, you need to ask them to stop the actions that frighten the puppy, calm him by stroking, and urge him closer to the person entering so that he is convinced that there is no threat from the outsider.

The goal of most dog breeders is to raise a dog that would become a good guard. If a puppy 3-4 months of age and older is indifferent to a stranger who has entered the apartment or meets him with joy, it is necessary to conduct several classes to develop his skills in proper behavior. To do this, you need to ask a friend in front of the apartment door not to knock, but rather energetically scrape the door. If the puppy is alert and starts to bark, it should be encouraged by exclaiming "Good!" and stroking. A similar behavior, only in a more pronounced form, should manifest itself when an outsider enters the apartment.

If these actions do not cause the desired reaction, it is necessary that an outsider stir up the puppy with sharp threatening actions. When the puppy is alert and begins to bark, an outsider should step back and, having shown his "fright," leave the apartment. The owner should reassure the puppy by stroking and exclaiming "Good!.."

The actions of an outsider in relation to the puppy should not be very harsh, not frightening. It is enough if the puppy shows a moderate offensive-defensive reaction, but one must not allow him to show cowardice.

It is categorically not recommended to arouse alertness and an active defensive reaction in a puppy by dressing in the clothing of its neighbors and acting threateningly on it. The puppy will quickly expose the owner by smell and other individual characteristics.

If puppies at the age of 3-5 months have little acquaintance with the environment due to insufficient physical development and lack of formation of behavioral reactions, they often exhibit a passive-defensive reaction in response to external stimuli, retreating, frightened, and trying to hide. Such a reaction is undesirable, so the puppy should be reassured and distracted by a game or treat. As a rule, this behavior of a puppy is not a manifestation of an innate and undecided passive-defensive reaction due to a weak type of higher nervous activity. This is a natural reaction to an unfamiliar external stimulus. With regular practice with the puppy, she will be replaced by a defensive reaction in an active form. If the passive-defensive reaction persists in the puppy despite the lessons, heredity should be "blamed" on this.

As a result of the upbringing, the puppy must learn what actions he will be encouraged by the treat and exclamation "Good!," and for which they will be punished. Punishment should be applied when the puppy tries to commit an unwanted action or immediately after it, having previously given the prohibiting command "No!."

For the upbringing and initial training of the puppy, a harness, a collar, a long and short leash, as well as bags for treats and toys are needed.

## Initial Training

First, consider the age characteristics of puppies and approaches to training each of the three age groups.

Puppies at the age of 1-3 months are taught to master and know the new members of his family, feeding, their place, cleanliness, nickname, harness and leash, approach to the owner ("Come!"), departure from the owner ("Take a walk!," "Go!"), the cessation of unwanted actions ("No!"), games with the owner and peers, and environmental irritants (for a walk).

Puppies easily develop positive skills associated with any activity and with difficult skills based on inhibitory reactions. To develop the necessary skills, it is recommended to use goodies.

At the age of 3–6 months, puppies continue to be accustomed to cleanliness, nickname, performance of the commands "Place!," "Come!," "Go!," "No!," games with the owner and peers, and environmental irritants. The puppy gets accustomed to a collar, leash, and a muzzle. They begin to work out the commands.

In contrast to 1-3-month-old animals, the necessary skills of 3-6-month-old puppies are developed in the process of one or another activity not only with the help of food (treats) but also with mechanical influences (palm pressure, light tension and jerking with a leash, etc.) Food (delicacy), as a rule, is used to reward the execution of the action.

At the age of 6-8 months. the puppy is taught to execute the commands better. He also understands how to overcome obstacles, move in settlements, behave in vehicles, and endurance. Games continue with the owner and peers and you need to take more walks.

During this period, the puppy is taught to execute commands given simultaneously with gestures, as well as separately. The training technique is becoming more complicated, the requirements for a puppy are increasing. For a clearer execution of commands, not only tension is allowed, but moderate jerking with a leash and palm presses on body parts (compulsion method). But, as before, all actions on the puppy should be gentle, as his body at this age has not yet been sufficiently formed.

In order for the command execution skills to meet the requirements of the general training course, it is necessary to gradually train the puppy to perform them without a leash. It is possible to teach a puppy to work without a leash only when he develops and consolidates skills when working with him on a leash on one or another action. Otherwise, the puppy will not only "learn nothing," but will also lose its previously acquired skills.

## Training for the owner and members of his family

The puppy gets used to the owner and members of his family in the process of constant communication with them. If a puppy is treated with care and does not allow any action that causes pain or timidity, then a good relationship is established and strengthened between it and others. The strongest contact should be made between the puppy and its owner. Therefore, the owner should be engaged in the maintenance and upbringing of the puppy, and the rest of the family members can take care of him in case of emergency (the owner's illness, etc.).

If, when the owner appears, the puppy runs up to him and starts to caress, jumps up, and barks maliciously, accompany him around the apartment or in the yard and try to start a game. If the owner leaves, he becomes anxious, sometimes whines, waits at the door until the necessary contact has been made. Yet, he should learn to live in the owner's absence and be part of the whole family. The point here is that dogs need a leader, and there can be only one!

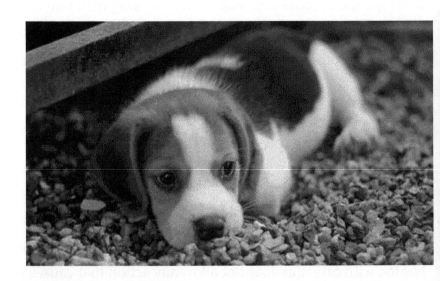

# Chapter 7

## Basics

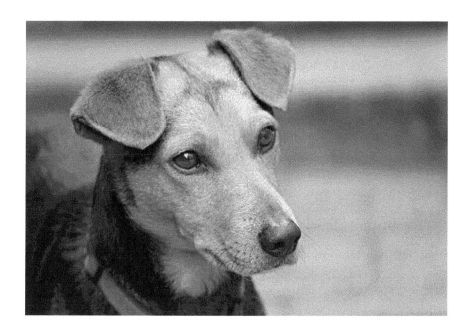

## Training for Feeding

Regular intake of food and water is a vital need. You do not need to train a puppy for this. When he was taken from his mother and transferred to another owner, he was already accustomed to various feeds. It is important to regularly feed and give water to the puppy, at the same time, observe the usefulness of the daily diet, following scientifically sound recommendations.

It is unacceptable to overfeed. In the first case, this will lead to a lag in growth and development. It will also disrupt the normal digestion process, impair appetite, and provoke obesity.

## Dishes for feeding

It is necessary to teach a dog to return to a place both in everyday life and with special training. The conditioned stimuli here are the command and gesture, the unconditional ones are an encouragement and a slight tug by the leash.

They begin to teach a puppy to his place from the first days of his appearance in the house. The place where the dog should lie is intended for resting the puppy, as well as for its temporary placement in cases where it interferes with people (cleaning the premises, eating, etc.).

Every time a puppy, having satiated or played enough, starts laying somewhere to rest, you need to pick it up, put it in its place and put it on the mat after the "Place!" command, then repeat the command and stroke it. At first, the puppy will usually try to get up and run away. In this case, holding him on the bedding, you should repeat the command "Place!" while stroking, and when he calms down, encourage him with an exclamation of "Good" while still stroking, and then move away. Even if the puppy has fallen asleep, this exercise can be completed. If he gets up and tries to lie down somewhere else, the exercise should be repeated. During the day, the exercise should be repeated 3-4 times.

Using this technique, a puppy is taught to leave according to the "Place!" command in cases when, during a meal by people, he will beg or start chasing a broom when cleaning an apartment.

It should be borne in mind that it is relatively easy to teach a puppy to execute a command when he is full or tired. It is much more difficult to do this when it is excited by the smell of food at the table or attracted by a broom or vacuum cleaner moving across the floor. In the first case, skills are easily developed in young, 1–2-month-old puppies, and in the second, in puppies who are 3–4 months of age or older. Gradually, your puppy will get used to the command.

You can also train the puppy at the age of 3–6 months. Do it as follows. When it is necessary to send a puppy, call him and take him to his place. Then repeat the command and put the puppy on the mat, after which you encourage it with an exclamation of "Good!," stroke, and leave. After the puppy lies down, call him and play with him a little. If after the command he does not go to the place, repeat the command in a more strict tone and carry him there. If this does not help, use a leash with a harness or collar. Take the puppy on command to its place on the leash, remove the harness or collar, put the puppy on the mat, repeat the command "Place!," and encourage with "Good!" with treats and strokes.

Gradually, after the action, you reduce the number of escorts and then send the puppy to the place without accompaniment. During the day, this exercise should be repeated 4-5 times.

At the age of 6–8 months, the "Place!" action is being worked out not only in the apartment but also in the yard.

The puppy is taken on a long leash, laid on the command "Place!" and put in front of him some object that would indicate his place. You then say the command a second time, move away from the puppy by 3-5 steps and turn to him. After a short pause, the puppy is called to yourself, encouraged, then you make such a gesture - you stretch their right-hand palm down to the height of the belt in the direction of the place that the puppy left, and lower them to the thigh of the right leg with a slight tilt of the body forward, at the same time giving the command "Place!" . At the same time, with your left hand, make several light jerks with a leash and go with the puppy to the designated place. At the same time, you release the puppy forward, accustoming them to move to the place on their own. While driving, you should repeat the "Place!" command 2-3 times. Leading the puppy to the subject, lay it and encourage. The exercise is repeated with short breaks 2-3 times.

If the puppy moves away from his place, the command should be given in a more strict tone, and if this does not help, the puppy should be taken to a place on a leash.

When the puppy develops the skill for the command and gesture, the "Place!" command after the gesture needs to be given less and less, and then be limited to one gesture. Then the puppy is sent to the place by command and gesture at the same time.

The skill is developed if the dog without a leash on the first command and the gesture of the owner (trainer) quickly and clearly returns to its original place from a distance of 15 ft, independently lays down no further than 1 ft from the subject (place), and maintains its position for up to 30 seconds.

## Accustoming to Cleaning and Washing

The puppy is taught to be cleaned and washed from an early age when it was taken from its mother and kept in the house or in the yard. Difficulties in the development of this skill do not arise if the puppy is taught to be washed and cleaned carefully, without causing pain and without scaring him. Cleaning will become a source of pleasant sensations for the puppy, and each time, he will be happy to run to the owner, having seen a brush or comb in his hand.

This applies equally to training a puppy to wash. It is necessary to carefully monitor the temperature of the water, especially if you use a hose with a mixer. There are times when warm water suddenly gives way to hot water and a puppy gets burned. After that, for many days only the noise of water flowing out of the hose will cause him fright and resistance to washing. Do not use water directly from hoses with such mixers for washing.

## Potty Training

A puppy is taught cleanliness from the first day of his appearance in the house. At the age of 3–6 months, high requirements are imposed on the cleanliness of puppies. Usually, by the age of 3 months, the puppy gets used to asking for a dump (excreta or pee) in a timely manner, but "doesn't stand it" quite often. Carried away by a game or some other activity, he still may not respond in a timely manner to the body's signals. Therefore, you need to regularly and timely watch your puppy. It should be noted that several dogs, including puppies, cannot get rid of urine in one go and do this several times.

It is best to bring the puppy out without waiting for him to ask. If the puppy's behavior becomes restless, he should be allowed to go immediately.

Particular attention should be paid to feeding. Poor quality products and stale food can cause digestion, in which case, the puppy will cause you trouble.

For your dog, especially at a younger age, let the process for taking a dump be regular and at a set time. Dogs are clean animals so, in a little while, it will naturally start to go there on their own.

# Nickname Training

The puppy gets used to the nickname quickly, within 3-4 days. The nickname is pronounced when you turn to the puppy during grooming, feeding, raising, initial and training. Therefore, you need to seriously make the choice for nicknames.

The nickname must match the puppy's gender. It should be short, simple, easily pronounced, and harmonious. You can't assign nicknames using human names, military ranks, nationality, names of states, or cities. The nickname should cause sympathy for the dog. Names discrediting an animal are inadmissible.

To teach a puppy a nickname during the day, clearly and loudly pronounce it. As soon as the puppy draws attention to it, he should be immediately encouraged by stroking and repeating the nickname. For each feeding, this is also used. Before feeding you take a feeder, pronounce the nickname, and after the reaction of the puppy, immediately put it in its place and feed the puppy. During feeding, the nickname is repeated 1-2 times.

It is especially important to develop the ability of a puppy to immediately respond to a nickname when it is distracted by something, such as toys, a bone, watches a cat, etc. For this, before each feeding, you wait until the puppy is distracted, pronounce its nickname and when he turns its attention, put the feeder and feed it. Do not forget to repeat the nickname 1-2 times.

After the puppy begins to respond to the nickname, to consolidate the developed skill, you need to encourage it daily by stroking whenever it draws its attention to the pronounced nickname, but gradually reduce the number of rewards. In the future, encouragement, especially a treat, is occasionally resorted to, as a rule, if the puppy stops responding or responds inconsistently to his nickname.

By the age of 3 months, the puppy gets used to the nickname, and in the future, this skill requires only consolidation and improvement. To this end, the puppy is periodically encouraged when he reacts to the nickname and is drawn attention to the owner. But dogs are encouraged less and less and replaced by an exclamation of "Good!" and stroking. When the puppy's ability to promptly respond to a nickname is developed, the need for such incentives disappears, as they are replaced by the pleasure that the puppy experiences when performing subsequent exercises (classes). For example, after the puppy reacts to the nickname and draws its attention to the owner, he takes him on a leash and takes him for a walk, which is a great encouragement for the puppy.

You turn to the puppy when he is distracted by something. Then the exercise is carried out in a complex: pronouncing the nickname, then give the command "Come!," and then "Place!," etc.

When accustoming a puppy to a nickname, it is not recommended to pronounce it too often. Pronouncing a nickname in front of each action too often can teach a puppy to execute commands only in combination with a nickname, which is unacceptable.

# Harness and Leash Training

You need to train your puppy to harness and leash from 2–2.5 months of age. Select the appropriate harness and adjust it so that it does not hang out and at the same time does not hamper the puppy's movements. After that, carefully, but rather quickly put on a puppy harness. If the puppy is worried and tries to get rid of it, he is calmed by stroking, distracted by a game, or a short run. If this does not help and the puppy will still be very worried, you need to remove the harness and allow him to run a little, and then put on the harness again. During the day, the exercise is repeated 3-4 times.

When the puppy begins to behave calmly with the worn harness during the walk, quickly and whenever possible, fasten the leash (shorten it) to the harness then again release it and lower it to the ground. After a 3-5-minute walk, take the leash in the left hand and, pulling it slightly, continue the walk. During the day, the exercise is repeated 4-5 times. The leash is designed to hold and control the puppy during walking and running. In the future, it is also used in developing skills for various actions.

The puppy needs to be calm about the leash. This usually happens as soon as the owner takes the leash in his hand and the puppy starts running around him, bouncing and showing other signs of joy. Therefore, it is wrong to use a leash to punish a puppy. To do this, use the rod and resort to it in case of emergency when other educational measures do not reach the goal. If you punish the puppy with a leash, even slightly, he will become afraid of it. With systematic abuse of the leash, the puppy starts to run away and hide from the owner every time he takes the leash in his hands.

At the same time, you cannot turn a leash into a toy, as many dog breeders often do. It is unacceptable that the puppy while playing with a leash, nibble it and pull it towards himself. In this case, the leash loses its value as a tool to discipline the puppy, especially when walking. The puppy quickly gets used to the harness and leash.

## Training for a Collar

A puppy is trained to a collar and leash from 3 months of age according to the method of training for a harness with a leash. By this time, the puppy's neck is sufficiently formed and strengthened, the collar, if used properly, does not cause pain and allows you to control the puppy. However, we must not forget that with a strong pull, the collar makes breathing difficult. Therefore, sharp pulls and jerks with a leash are unacceptable. If the task of finer control of the leash is not set for the development of certain skills, it is more expedient to use not a leash, but a harness.

# Muzzle Training

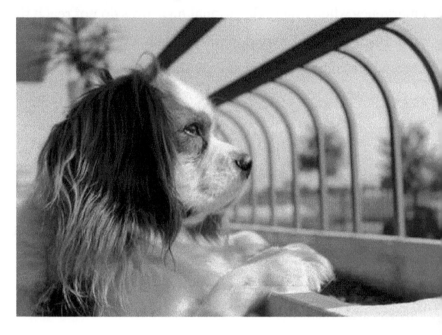

Training your puppy for a muzzle can start at 4 months of age. The most convenient is a muzzle where front consists of a solid piece of leather or leatherette with holes for air. It allows the dog to keep its mouth open if necessary and makes breathing easier. In the warm season, a mesh metal muzzle is convenient.

The muzzle is selected in accordance with the size of the puppy' face, and if necessary, fit it so that it does not particularly hamper the puppy and does not hang out. During a walk with a puppy on a leash, you need to stop, show him the muzzle so that he can smell it, and with a careful, but quick movement of your dominant hand put on and fasten the muzzle, after which you can continue the walk. If the puppy makes an attempt to break free from the muzzle, you can run around with it and calm it down with stroking. To distract the puppy, you can give the commands "Sit!," etc. After 2-3 minutes, the muzzle is removed and after a short break, the exercise is repeated 2-3 times. In the future, you need to increase the puppy's stay in the muzzle.

## Learning to Approach the Owner (Trainer)

To approach the owner by the command "Come!," the puppy is taught immediately after establishing contact with him and being accustomed to the nickname and place. This skill is very important for the owner of the puppy and adult dog, so its development should be treated with due attention. The conditioned irritants are the "Come!" command and gesture, while the unconditional ones are food, easy pulling of the leash, and stroking.

During a walk without a leash, the puppy will periodically disappear from the field of view of the owner, especially in places overgrown with dense shrubs. Usually, a puppy watches the owner, but if he finds a bone or a fish head, then he can forget about everything for a while. Therefore, it is necessary to ensure that the puppy, wherever he is and no matter what he does, immediately runs up to the owner at the command "Come!"

To break away from an interesting object (strong irritant) and run to the owner, the puppy has to overcome strong "research" instincts. Therefore, it's enough if he leaves the subject and goes to the owner by the command "Come!," even if repeated. At first he will do it slowly, but after repeated exercises, he will come up faster.

To develop a clear, sustainable skill for the action, the owner requires patience, perseverance, and passion. A puppy and an adult dog who did not master this skill will bring the owner a lot of problems and troubles, especially during the estrus period in bitches, since it is very difficult to restrain the manifestation of the sexual instinct in dogs.

It is possible to achieve the reliability and clarity of the "Come!" command from the puppy only if the action is perceived as a signal for further encouragement, accompanied by pleasant sensations (a game, exclamation "Good!," or a treat). Therefore, the puppy is taught to carry out the command with the help of food (goodies).

When you start feeding, you take a feeder, pronounce the nickname and, as soon as the puppy draws attention to it, you give the command "Come!" and then put the feeder in its place. Seeing that the puppy is running up, the owner gives the command "Come!," and when he runs up, encourage him with an exclamation of "Good!," stroke and gives food. This is done before the start of each feeding. First, you call a puppy in the same room and watch the action, and then do it when he is in another room, in the corridor and will be busy with something (a toy, etc.). Thus, you act on the principle "from simple to complex."

After 4–5 days of training, begin to work out the "Come!" action, taking the puppy out of the house. When the puppy moves away from the owner by 7-8 steps during the walk, you pronounce his nickname. As soon as the puppy pays attention to it, give a "Come!" command. When the puppy runs to the owner, he is encouraged by exclaiming "Good!," and stroke. During one walk, the exercise is repeated 4-5 times.

Often, especially in the early days of classes, a puppy may not respond to its nickname and command. In this case, the nickname is repeated louder, and when the puppy draws attention to it, even louder and in an imperative tone you give the command "Come!," but in no case shout. Then you show the puppy a treat and, if this does not work on him, you call him his nickname, run a little to the side or sit down. As a rule, this causes interest in the puppy, and he runs up to the owner. Immediately encourage him with an exclamation of "Good!" and a stroke. Such a "maneuver" is also used if the puppy comes to the owner by the command "Come!" but too slowly.

Some puppies, despite all the efforts of the owner, poorly execute the command or even refuse to fulfill it. In this case, resort to the method of coercion, although it is undesirable for puppies. It should be used very carefully and only for older puppies. The puppy is taken on a long leash and, when it moves away from the owner, you pronounce the nickname and give the command "Come!," then, carefully pulling the leash, slowly pull the puppy closer to yourself, repeating the command 2-3 times. One must strive not to hurt the puppy. As soon as he approaches the owner, he is encouraged by the exclamation of "Good!," and some stroking.

Repeating the exercises, gradually complicate the training. Periodically give the command "Come!" without first pronouncing a nickname. This command is given when the puppy is carried away by something and hides from the owner. Gradually increase the distance between the owner and the puppy at the time of command. However, you can't complicate the task too much and make it impossible for the puppy. It should be remembered that the requirement of an immediate, trouble-free, and energetic approach should be increased gradually, as the initial skills are developed and the puppy's age increases.

At the age of 3–6 months, the implementation of the "Come!" action continues to be consolidated and improved, allowing moderate coercion (mechanical impact). If the puppy does not fit on command, he, having given the command, is gently pulled up with a long leash, and then encouraged with an exclamation of "Good!" along with stroking. The exercise is repeated 3-4 times.

The task is complicated gradually. The puppy is called up on the command "Come!" when he is distracted or went away somewhere. The distance between the owner and the puppy is increased. At the same time, each time the nickname is preliminarily pronounced to attract the puppy's attention, and when he reacts, give the command.

At the age of 6–8 months, the "Come!" action is being worked out and improved with a long leash. If the puppy, after the command and showing the goodies, does not answer the command, then repeat it more strictly and easily pull the leash, pulling the puppy to yourself and repeating the command 1-2 times. When the puppy is near the owner, you encourage him with an exclamation of "Good!," and stroking daintily. One must try not to hurt the puppy. After a short break, the exercise is repeated. In subsequent classes, it is necessary to ensure that the puppy, on command, goes to the owner without the help of a leash, and does not come up, but runs up. Encouragement should be slowly phased out.

After the puppy gets used to running up to the owner by the command "Come!," then begin to practice the reaction to the gesture. When the puppy runs away from the owner on a long leash, then pronounce its nickname to attract his attention and make such a gesture - raise the right hand to the side to the shoulder level with the palm down and quickly lower it to the thigh of the right leg, then give the command "Come!." A puppy is encouraged by an exclamation of "Good!," stroking and a treat. The exercise is repeated with small interruptions 3-4 times.

In the future, you should call the puppy with a command and a gesture at the same time, but then periodically resort to either one action or one gesture, ensuring that the gesture becomes equivalent to the puppy's command.

If the puppy is reluctant to respond to the gesture, it can be activated by showing a treat in the right hand or running back a few steps.

Also in the future, the puppy is trained on the command "Come!" to run to the owner, bypassing him on the right and behind, and to sit at his left foot. To do this, pronounce the nickname of the puppy, make a gesture, and pronounce the command "Come!." The running puppy is shown a treat in the right hand, taken away behind the back and, shifting to the left hand, prompts the puppy to follow the owner after the treat to the back and go to the left side. When the puppy is at the left leg, the treat should be shifted to the right hand and raised up and a little back, forcing the puppy to sit down. If he does not sit down, then perform the command "Sit!." The exercise is repeated 3-4 times, achieving faster execution of the command.

This skill is considered developed if the dog from any distance, at different times and in the presence of distracting stimuli, by the first command and gesture quickly runs up to the trainer (owner), runs around him on the right behind, stops at his left foot, and sits down.

## Learning to Transition to a Free State

Departing from the owner by the command "Walk!," the puppy is taught after he is accustomed to carrying out the command "Come!." The conditioned command is the "Walk!" command and the gesture, while the unconditioned are the animal's internal natural needs for freedom.

During the walk, you unfasten the leash, give the command "Walk!" and drag the puppy along with a small run to make it run forward. After the puppy walks a little, he is called to yourself and encouraged by stroking. In the future, having given the command, you reduce the run, and subsequently send it forward at the command "Walk!," with you remaining in one place. During the day, the exercise should be repeated 4-5 times

As the initial skills are developed, the exercise is complicated. The puppy is sent further away, increasing the time of his stay in a free state, but do not abuse the complications.

At the age of 3–6 months, the skill of completing the action is consolidated and improved. This success is a reward for the puppy and therefore does not require special efforts on the part of the owner. However, its timely and clear implementation should be sought. During the day, the exercise is repeated 2-3 times. The puppy's movement route in a free state and the duration of the walk gradually increases.

At the age of 6–8 months, the "Walk!" action is practiced on a long leash after developing skills for the "Come!" action and a gesture. The puppy is placed at the left foot, pronouncing its nickname and quickly moving the right-hand palm down towards the desired movement of the puppy, then lowering it to the thigh with a slight tilt of the body forward, giving the command "Walk!." Following this, run forward, dragging the puppy. The exercise is repeated 3-4 times. Gradually, the puppy is given the opportunity to run back alone. A command after a gesture is served less and less, then they are limited to one gesture, reinforcing it with a command only occasionally.

The skill is considered developed if the puppy immediately goes to the free state under any conditions and from any position by the first command "Walk!" and the gesture of the trainer (owner), but does not run too far.

## Learning to Stop a Certain Act or Action

This skill is necessary so that the owner (trainer), with the help of the action, can timely stop the unwanted action of the puppy (dog) or attempts to commit them. The "Stop!" command serves as a conditioned stimulus, unconditional - at first a blow with a rod, then a jerk with a leash. For an adult dog, a strict collar jerk is sometimes used. However, you only reach the goal if it is served at the moment when the puppy (adult dog) begins an undesirable action.

At the age of 1-3 months, the puppy is taught to stop unwanted actions on the command "Stop!" carefully so as not to slow down its activity, the natural desire to run and play. It should be remembered that up to 2.5-3 months of age, the puppy easily develops positive skills associated with any activity, for example, the commands "Come!" and "Walk!," but it is still difficult to develop inhibitory reactions. Therefore, at the age of 1-3 months, resorting to mechanical stress is impossible.

You can wean a puppy from evil deeds using the method of distraction and switching his attention to another occupation, for example, a game. To distract the puppy from unwanted actions, you can pronounce his nickname, give the command "Come!" and show a treat. As soon as the puppy runs to the owner, you need to play with him and only after a while encourage a treat so that he does not consider that he is encouraged for unwanted actions.

Puppies at the age of 1-3 months cannot be punished. An exception may be cases if repeated attempts to distract him from unwanted actions were unsuccessful. Then the puppy can be lightly hit with a twig on the back and at the same time say the command "Stop!." This should be done as soon as the puppy tries to perform an undesirable action, and only with puppies 2.5-3 months of age.

Puppies of 3-6 months of age are taught to stop unwanted actions on the command "Stop!." During this age period, the requirements for them are gradually increasing.

When developing this skill, each time the puppy tries to produce an undesirable action, you say the command "Stop!"

(conditioned stimulus) with threatening intonation, which is immediately reinforced by mechanical action (unconditional stimulus). The "Stop!" command and mechanical impact should not scare the puppy. Exercise throughout the day is repeated 3-4 times.

When the puppy develops the initial skill for the "Stop!" action and begins to fulfill it, it is possible to confine itself to one action (the word "Stop!") and apply an unconditional reinforcing stimulus so that the developed skill does not fade.

At the age of 6–8 months, the conditions for practicing the "Stop!" action is becoming more complicated, and requirements for the puppy are increasing. The main task in this period is to achieve a clearer response to the command to stop unwanted actions. The puppy is taught not to pick up bones and other food debris from the ground and not to take food that outsiders offer.

The "Stop!" command and jerks are used with a leash in order to wean the puppy from pouncing on people, vehicles, and barking during walks.

## Learning to play with a host and peers

You can teach a puppy to play with the owner just a few days after he gets used to the situation and his master. To do this, use toys that are periodically thrown to the floor, short runs, etc. Games with the owner should compensate for games with peers. During the game, you need to try to imitate the actions of other puppies: to tip the puppy on his back, etc. but this must be done carefully, trying not to hurt the puppy, and for a short time. To develop a puppy's sense of self-confidence, courage, perseverance, and initiative, it is useful to periodically imitate his victory over the owner.

Other family members can play with the puppy, but carefully and for a short time. However, in no case can you turn a puppy into a living toy, as this will lead to overwork and impaired appetite.

Games with peers are useful for the physical development of the puppy and for his education. Nothing can fully replace his games with peers. An indispensable condition for this should be the health of puppies, approximately the same age. The owner must watch the game.

The duration of the game needs to be regulated and gradually increased. Where puppies play, there should not be objects that could injure them. After each game, the puppy must be laid for rest.

For 3–8-month-old puppies, playing with the owner and peers should be practiced daily if possible, gradually increasing their duration and intensity using various toys.

## Learning to walk

A puppy is taught to walk after it has become accustomed to the owner. Walking with puppies at the age of 1-3 months should be cautious because according to their physical development and state of higher nervous activity, they are still not formed and strengthened and the increased stress for them is too great.

Walking is needed not only to improve health but also to gain life experience, adapt to environmental conditions, develop the right response to various, including strong, external stimuli (strangers, animals, vehicles, etc.). During a walk with a puppy on a harness and a leash periodically, you need to stop, give him the opportunity to get acquainted with various objects, allow him to sniff them, etc.

Every time a puppy is frightened of something, he needs to be reassured by stroking, taking a walk and bringing him back to the object so that he is convinced of the absence of danger. To do this, periodically use a treat.

In quiet places where nothing threatens the puppy, you can unfasten the leash and provide the opportunity to run free. This helps the puppy develop an initiative when familiarizing himself with surrounding objects and smells, differentiating them (recognizing, distinguishing), he learns to calmly and correctly respond to various stimuli, avoiding danger. However, you cannot weaken the attention to the puppy and the environment, you need to take the puppy on a leash in a timely manner if a car or some other danger appears.

You should not overwork the puppy with long, unbearable walks for him, or bring him to a state where he becomes indifferent and ceases to be interested in surrounding objects. It is especially necessary to ensure that the puppy does not go out of sight of the owner, since at any time he may need help.

Walking with puppies older than 3 months is carried out daily, gradually increasing the time and length. They are connected on a leash with a collar. In quiet places, the leash is unfastened and gives the puppy the opportunity to walk freely. It is not recommended to walk with him in the immediate vicinity of vehicles that make loud noises. If the puppy is frightened, he needs to be reassured by stroking and distracting him with a treat. After a while, approach the object that scared him again to make him sure that there is no threat.

# Occupation next to the owner

To train a puppy to move next to the owner by the command "Near!" begins at the age of 3–6 months after he is accustomed to a collar and leash. The conditioned stimuli are command and gesture, while the unconditioned ones are stroking and a leash with a collar.

In a quiet place, the puppy is taken on a short leash and placed near the left foot. With your left hand, hold the leash 30–35 cm from the collar so that it can easily move in a bent form. With your right hand, hold the rest of the leash in the middle, after putting the loop on your hand above the dog. Then give the command "Near" and immediately pull the leash forward, then carry the puppy next to you. Each time he makes an attempt to move away or fall behind, then give the command "Near!" and hold him by pulling the leash (not in a jerk!). Then weaken the tension of the leash, allowing the puppy to move freely near the left leg.

If the puppy is anxious during movement, whisk him along while stroking with your left hand. In the early days, the puppy can be very anxious. In such cases, you need to stop, calm him by stroking, and resume movement on the command "Next!." The puppy should not be allowed to move more than 0.5 ft away. The exercise is repeated 3-4 times during the day.

The length of the route is gradually increased. In no case should you allow a jerk with a leash (this can only be done with 6-month-old puppies). In this exercise, at this stage, it is important to ensure that the puppy moves close to the left of the owner by the command "Near!."

When practicing this command with puppies aged 6–8 months, jerking with a leash are allowed. The puppy is placed at the left foot. They are given the command "Next!" and at the same time, as they move forward with a jerk of a short leash, carry him along. The puppy's attempts to run ahead or move to the side are stopped by a jerk of the leash. Once the puppy is in the correct position, he is encouraged by an exclamation of "Good!" and you then continue to move. The leash tension can be loosened, causing the puppy to make a mistake so that you can correct it where necessary.

Gradually complicate the exercise by changing the speed of movement and practicing turns to the sides and around (to the right).

To develop a puppy's ability to walk on a short leash, you can put him near your left leg, clap your thigh, give the command "Next!," make a slight jerk with the leash and at the same time begin to move. Gradually, the command ("Next!") and jerking with the leash after the gesture is done less and less and is limited only to the gesture.

The skill is considered developed if a dog without a leash on the first command quickly occupies the correct position at the left foot of the owner (trainer) and retains it for a long time without any changes in direction and pace of movement.

## The "Sit!" command

To train a puppy to sit on the "Sit!" command, you should begin at the age of 3 months, when the initial skills for the commands "Come!" and "Near!" have been developed. The conditioned stimuli are the "Sit!" command and the gesture, while the unconditioned ones are a treat, a pressure on the lower back, and a slight jerk with a leash.

You call the puppy to yourself so that it becomes near the owner's left foot, call the nickname, and give the command "Sit!" The puppy will approach the treat, raise his head and sit down, so it is more convenient for him to watch the treat in your hand. If the puppy tries to take possession of the treat, it is held by the collar so that it does not pounce, but raises its head. As soon as the puppy sits down, it is encouraged by an exclamation of "Good!" and strokes. After short breaks, the exercise is repeated 2-3 times.

In 4–5 days after the initial skills of the "Sit!" action has been developed, proceed to work out the action in the yard and in places where there are no strong distracting irritants.

At the age of 6-8 months, the command is further trained on a short leash. The puppy is placed at the left foot and is turned halfway to you. You then take the leash with the right hand about 60 mm from the collar, and put the left hand on the puppy's lower back closer to the sacrum, with your thumb to yourself. Then give the "Sit!" command, press the lower back with the left hand, and at the same time, pull the leash up and a little back with the right hand. As soon as the puppy sits down, is encouraged by exclamation of "Good!" and stroke. After short breaks, the exercise is repeated 2-3 times.

When the puppy develops initial skills with the "Sit!" command you can proceed to work out the action at a distance of several steps. The puppy is placed on a short leash opposite the owner a a distance of 2–2.5 steps, pronouncing its nickname to attract his attention, and giving the command "Sit!." As soon as the puppy sits down, it is encouraged by an exclamation of "Good!" and some stroking. After short breaks, the exercise is repeated 2-3 times.

If the puppy does not execute the command, it should be repeated more strictly. If after this it is not completed, you need to go to the puppy, give the command "Sit!" and apply left-hand pressure on the lower back and pulling the leash with your right hand up and a little back to make the puppy sit down. Then he is encouraged by the exclamation of "Good!" and some stroking. They stand the puppy, move away from him by 2–2.5 steps, turn to him and give the command "Sit!." After holding for 5-7 seconds, the puppy is summoned towards you and encouraged.

If the puppy moves to the owner without you calling him, then quickly approach him, take him with the leash and make him sit on command. If the action fails, use the leash and press the lower back with your hand, as described above.

To develop a puppy's skill of sitting by a gesture, it can be done as follows. The puppy is laid opposite you in 1.5–2 steps. Then take a leash into the left hand and pull it slightly, then quickly stretch the right hand to the side at shoulder level, bend at the elbow, giving the forearm a vertical position (palm forward), lower it to the thigh of the right leg and give the command "Sit!." After the command is completed, you need to go to the puppy and encourage him with an exclamation of "Good!" and some stroking. After some time, the exercise is repeated 2-3 times. Gradually, the vocal command is served less and less, and then they are limited only by a gesture, occasionally reinforcing it with a vocal command.

In the future, the puppy is seated by the "Sit!" command, while simultaneously making a gesture, but this is periodically carried out only by command or only by a gesture. The skill is considered developed if the dog clearly, quickly and without fail from various positions and under any conditions, sits by the first command and the gesture of the owner (trainer), being at a distance of up to 15 ft from you, and retains this position until the next command with an endurance of up to 15 seconds.

## Learning to "go to bed"

The puppy is taught to go to the "Lie!" command at the age of 3 months, immediately after the initial skills for the "Sit!" command has been developed. The conditioned stimuli are the "Lie!" command and gesture, while the unconditioned ones are a delicacy, pressure on the withers, and a leash with a collar.

You need to put the puppy at the left foot, make a half-turn to the left, give the nickname and give the command "Lie!," and after that, bringing the treat to his face in your right hand. Bending down, gently lower the treat down and forward. Rushing for a treat, the puppy will bend down and lie down. Then he is encouraged by the exclamation of "Good!" and a treat, while simultaneously pressing the withers with your left hand. After short breaks, the exercise is repeated 2-3 times.

In 4–5 days after the development of initial skills, classes can be continued in the yard, avoiding strong distracting irritants.

The command "Lie!" with 6-8-month-old puppies is practiced on a short leash. The puppy is seated at the left leg, turned halfway to you. Then take the leash in your right hand, and put the left hand on the withers. Then they give the command "Lie!." Press the withers with your left hand and at the same time make a long jerk with a leash down and a little forward. As soon as the puppy lies down, he is encouraged by exclaiming "Good!," and some stroking. If he tries to get up, you need to give the command again in a more rigorous tone and press the withers with your left hand, holding him in a "lie" position for 7-10 seconds. After some time, the exercise should be repeated 2-3 times.

After the puppy develops initial skills, the "Lie!" command will proceed to its development at a distance of several steps. The puppy on a short leash needs to be planted opposite you at a distance of 1.5–2 steps, pronounce the nickname and give the command "Lie!." As soon as the puppy lies down, he is encouraged by exclaiming "Good!," and with stroking. After short breaks, the exercise is repeated 2-3 times.

If the puppy does not execute the command, it must be repeated in a more strict tone. If even then it will not be fulfilled, you need to go to the puppy, give the command and, pushing the withers with your left hand and jerking the leash with your right hand down and slightly forward, make him lie down. After this, the puppy is encouraged with an exclamation of "Good!," some stroking, and a treat. Then, again, retreat 1.5–2 steps, turn to him and make him lie down with the command "Lie!." After 7-10 seconds of lying down, the puppy is summoned towards yourself and encouraged with an exclamation of "Good!," and some stroking. If he begins to move without your call, you need to quickly approach him, take him with the leash to its place and make the dog lie down with the command. If necessary, use the leash and hand pressure on the withers.

To develop the puppy's ability to go to bed by a gesture, you can follow the next procedures. The puppy is seated opposite in 1.5–2 steps. Take the leash into the left hand, pull it slightly and raise the right hand palm down forward to shoulder level, then quickly lower it to the hip. A little later, give the command "Lie!." When the puppy lies down, he needs to be encouraged. The exercise is repeated 2-3 times. Gradually, the command after the gesture is served less and less, and then limited to only the gesture.

The skill is considered developed if the dog in any conditions by the first command or the gesture of the trainer (owner), being at a distance of up to 5 ft from him, clearly and without fail, takes the lying position from any other and remains there until the next command up to 15 seconds.

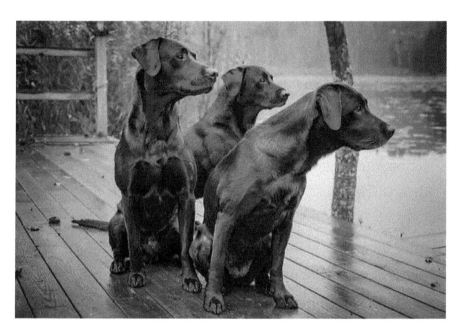

## Learning to Stand

The puppy is trained to stand on the command "Stand!" at 3 months of age after developing basic skills for the commands "Sit!" and "Lie!." The "Stand!" command and a gesture serve as conditioned stimuli; the unconditional stimuli are raising the puppy under the stomach with your left hand, a treat, and a light jerk with a leash.

The puppy is placed at your left leg and you make half a turn to him. Then, call the puppy's nickname and give the command "Stand!." Afterword, with light pressure with your left hand under his stomach, make him stand up. As soon as the puppy gets up, he is encouraged by the exclamation of "Good!," and some stroking. After short breaks, the exercise is repeated 2-3 times. If the puppy, rising, tries to move, it is held with the right hand on the collar.

In 4–5 days after developing the initial skills for the "Stand!" action, then begin to practice this exercise in the yard, avoiding strong irritants.

After the puppy learns to execute the commands "Sit!," "Lie!" And "Stand!" without the use of goodies and the influence of his hand, you can start complex exercises, periodically changing the order of commands. As skills are consolidated, food and mechanical effects should be used only occasionally so that thes skills do not fade away, but are maintained and consolidated. If the puppy does not execute the command, it is repeated more strictly. To attract the attention of the puppy, distracted at the time of the command, pronounce his nickname first, and then repeat the command.

With 6-8-month-old puppies, the "Stand!" action is practiced using a short leash. The puppy is planted near the left leg, then turn halfway to it, and give the command "Stand!." Then, with the left hand, brought under the stomach, it is forced to stand. In this case, the tension of the leash is held. When the puppy stands up, he should be encouraged. If he tries to sit down or lie down without a command, the "Stand!" command must be repeated in a more rigorous tone and with your left hand brought under his stomach, and also with his right hand to hold him from it for 7-10 seconds. The exercise should be repeated 2-3 times. Then practice the skill at a distance of several steps.

Developing a puppy's ability to stand by gesture can be as follows. The puppy is seated opposite in 1.5–2 steps. Take the leash with your left hand and pull it slightly. To make a gesture, wave your right hand, slightly bent at the elbow, palm up, forward to the level of the belt, lower them to the thigh of the right leg and a little later give the command "Stand!." As soon as the puppy gets up, he is encouraged. After a short break, the exercise is repeated 2-3 times. Gradually, the voice command is served less and less, and then they are limited only by a gesture, reinforcing it with a "Stand!" only occasionally. In the future, put the puppy on command and gesture at the same time.

The skill is considered developed if the dog, by the first

command and the gesture of the trainer (owner), from any position in any conditions at a distance of up to 15 ft, clearly and without fail adopts a standing position without a leash, and retains it until the next command up to 15 seconds.

# Chapter 8
## Intermediate Skills

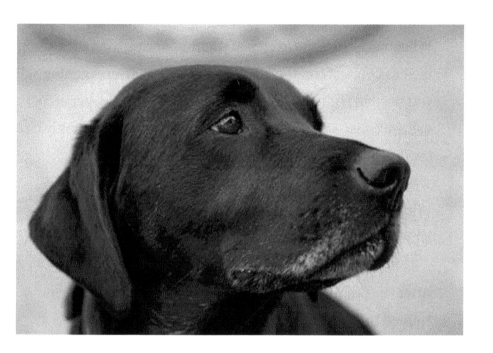

## Staircases and Ladders

The puppy begins to be taught to walk up the stairs at the age of 3 months on a short leash and harness. He needs to be brought to the stairs, put on the left, and given the command "Forward!." You need to start training carefully so as not to scare the puppy. If he is afraid to go down the stairs, you need to pull him slightly and make him interested in something. Pulling the leash with the left hand and holding the treat in the right, push it as if inviting to follow the movement of the hand. The puppy will try to grab the treat and follow you. After overcoming several steps, you need to encourage him by going down.

When mastering the exercise, you first need to drive the puppy next to yourself (on the left or behind you). Strengthening skills, you need to climb and go down the stairs with steeper steps, using a collar and a leash. The puppy must independently rise (or descend) at the command "Forward!."

With puppies aged 6–8 months, you can develop skills for climbing stairs with steeper steps and longer lengths.

After the puppy learns to walk the stairs confidently, he is trained to overcome low ladders using the same methodology. However, moving away from the ground, the puppy experiences anxiety and fear in the first days of classes, so that when lifting, and especially during the descent, it must be supported by a leash and encouraged by stroking.

After the puppy learns to walk through the staircase on a short leash next to the owner, you can start training without a leash. The puppy is planted in front of the staircase at the owner's left foot and the right hand is extended, palm down, toward the stairs, then lowered to the thigh with a slight tilt of the body forward, giving the command "Forward!." Following this, the puppy should be encouraged. The exercise is repeated 2-3 times.

The exercise is complicated using ladders of more complex structures. The skill is considered developed if the dog, on the first command and gesture, independently overcomes the ladder.

## Overcoming barriers

The skill of overcoming various obstacles disciplines the puppy and contributes to its physical development. While overcoming a barrier and continuous set of barriers the "Barrier!" action and "Forward!" command are used together. While overcoming the obstacles, the command, as well as the gesture, serve as the unconditioned stimulus. A treat and a toy — serve as conditioned stimuli.

Overcome obstacles, the puppy is trained from 3 months of age. Start with low barriers. Bring the puppy to a low obstacle (0.3 to 0.8 ft), then give the command "Forward!" and, stepping over it, carry it along (for example, with the help of a toy), allowing it to rest its paws on the obstacle. After overcoming the obstacles, the puppy is encouraged. The exercise is repeated several times. Strengthening the skill, you need to reduce the encouragement of treats and gradually increase the height of the obstacle. Make it a solid obstacle (so that the puppy does not crawl from below), he can be taught to jump by throwing a toy.

At the command "Forward!," the puppy learns to overcome the obstacle by jumping and leaning on top with its paws. Overcoming an unsupported jump must be practiced by the command "Barrier!." In order not to injure the puppy's paws, you need to put a light rail on two pegs on top, which he can first knock down. We need to make it clear that it is better not to lean on the rail. Stepping over the rail, drag the puppy behind it again at the command "Barrier!" and pull him up a little with the leash so that he does not lean with his paws. After overcoming the obstacles, you need to encourage the dog with an exclamation of "Good!" and a treat. In the future, treats need to be less and less.

When this exercise is completed, you can unfasten the leash. You can't increase the height of the obstacle all the time, as the puppy can injure itself, get scared, and this will permanently discourage him from jumping. For a 4-month-old puppy, the obstacle should not exceed 0.8 ft, while for a 5-month-old puppy, 1 – 1.5 ft.

It is easier to jump the puppy through the ditch, but its width should not exceed the indicated height by more than 10 cm.

Through the ditches, you need to train him to jump by the command "Forward!."

At the age of 6–8 months, the puppy is taught to overcome obstacles using the same technique. At the same time, the height of vertical and horizontal obstacles are gradually increased. He is placed without a leash, then give the command "Barrier!." As soon as the puppy overcomes the obstacle, he is encouraged. The exercise is repeated 1-2 times.

For unsupported high jumps, athletic barriers of 1.5 ft high are used for 6-month-old puppies and up to 2 ft for 7-month-old puppies. The length of ditches and other horizontal obstacles should be 10 cm longer than the height of vertical obstacles. To overcome horizontal obstacles use the "Forward!" command.

The puppy is taught to overcome obstacles by a gesture - stretch your right hand palm down in the direction of the obstacle, then lower them to the thigh with a slight tilt of the body forward. First, the gesture is used with the command, then the vocal call is served less and less. In the future, simultaneously use the command "Barrier!" or "Forward!" and a gesture. The skill is considered developed if a dog without a leash, on the first command and gesture, successfully overcomes with an unsupported jump any obstacles up to 3 ft high (barrier, fence) and 5 ft wide (ditch), without touching them.

# Movement on a log

A puppy at the age of 3 months is taught to walk on a log at the command "Forward!." To do this, the puppy should be located to the left of the owner at the beginning of a rather thick border or log (the log should be square or hewn from above and from below). First, you need to teach your puppy to walk on a log lying on the ground. Holding the puppy on the left with the right hand behind the harness, and with the right - under the belly from the bottom, lead him along the log, repeating the command "Forward"! After the puppy walks through the length of the log, you need to encourage him and give a treat.

When the puppy learns to walk on the log with support, you need to ensure it can start by itself. After that, you can start training on a round log. It is necessary to ensure that the puppy does not jump from the log without completing the exercise. The training should be fixed by replacing the harness with a collar, and then unfasten the leash.

Then you need to go to a log set at a low height. During training, the owner should hold the puppy by the leash close to the collar. Starting the log and repeating the command "Forward!," you need to slightly pull the leash in front of the puppy and, supporting it under the stomach, lead forward. After the puppy leaves the log, it should be encouraged.

If the puppy shows fear and it is difficult to bring him to the log, you can interest him with a treat. It is necessary to bring him to the log and, having given the command "Forward!," to carry on for a treat. The puppy will move for a treat and rise to the log. When he descends from the log to the ground, you need to give him a treat, accompanied by the encouragement "Good!." Gradually, you need to be limited only to encouragement and stroking.

For 6 to 8-month-old puppies, the length of the log is increased. The puppy is taught to overcome the log in a gesture - you extend the right hand palm down towards the log, then lower it to the thigh with a slight tilt of the body forward. First, the gesture is used with the vocal command, then this is served less and less. In the future, use the "forward" command and gesture at the same time. After fixing the skill, the exercise is complicated. To do this, send the puppy to the log from various positions.

The skill is considered developed if the dog flies up the log, moves along it, and descends without jumping off prematurely.

# Traffic in settlements

The movement in settlements of a 3-month-old puppy is taught first on a harness and then in a collar using a short leash. The first classes are held in quiet, less crowded places, and then they move to more crowded places loaded with vehicles. The main task of the exercises is to train the puppy to calmly react to irritants, including strong ones, without being distracted by them, without running out onto the roadway, all the time being at the owner's left foot.

Before starting the movement, the puppy is placed near the left leg and on a leash. Movement with a puppy in such areas is started by the command "Near!" and is performed according to the described methodology (accustoming to occupying a position near the owner).

In urban conditions, puppies are taught to walk only on sidewalks. As soon as he tries to get off the sidewalk to the carriageway, they give the command "Near!" and pull the leash without stopping the movement. Crossing the road at a pedestrian crossing, give the command "Next!."

The puppy's attempts to pounce on other animals, people, and vehicles are stopped by the "Stop!" command and a slight jerk o the leash.

# Chapter 9

## Advanced Skills

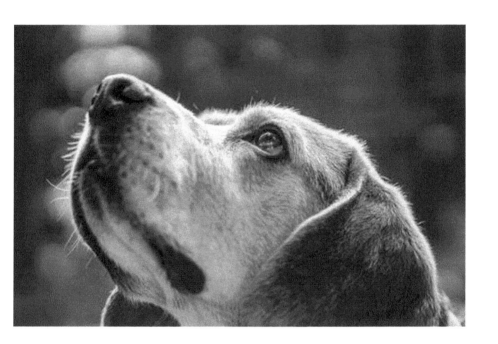

## Learning to Crawl

The "Crawl!" command can be taught to a 7-month-old puppy on a short leash. The conditioned irritants are the "Crawl!" command and the gesture, the unconditioned ones — pressing the withers, treats, and light jerks with its leash.

Choose a flat area free of objects that could injure or hurt your puppy, preferably covered in grass. The trainer lies on his right side, leaning on the elbow of his right hand, and puts the puppy to his left. He takes the leash in his right hand, puts the puppy down with some pressure on the withers, gives the command "Crawl!" and, starting to crawl, at the same time makes light jerks with his leash forward, prompting the puppy to crawl. If the puppy tries to rise, it must be held by pressing the left hand on the withers and at the same time give the command "Crawl!" When the puppy begins to crawl, he is encouraged. The distance is gradually increased from 1.5–2 ft to 5 ft.

When the puppy learns to crawl next to the trainer, go to the next stage. Lay the puppy on the command "Lie!" and lay an object or treat 2-3 m away from him. Then approach the puppy and give the command "Crawl!," holding it at the withers with your left hand, preventing it from getting up and pushing forward. As soon as he crawls to the right place, he is encouraged. If he doesn't want to crawl and lays on his back, then put him between the feet, not allowing him to turn over, and, taking the collar, make him crawl forward with light twitches, giving the command "Crawl!" at the same time. Puppy's attempts to crawl are always encouraged.

The skill is considered developed if the puppy crawls quickly and without fail along with the owner (trainer), as well as independently, to a distance of up to 1 5 in trouble-free terrain.

## Feed Rejection

This skill will protect the dog from attempts to poison it by intruders, not to be distracted by various types of food during work and not to pick up food waste from the ground. The "Stop!" command serves as a conditioned stimulus; the unconditional one is a jerk with a leash or a blow with a rod.

In the first lessons, the dog is taught not to eat food without the permission of the trainer. The feeder stands in front of the dog, its attempts to start eating are stopped by the command "Stop!" and holding the collar. After 5-10 seconds, the command "Eat" is given and the dog is allowed to start eating. Gradually, the exposure time is increased to 1 minute.

After this, the dog is taught not to take food from outsiders. In the first lessons, the dog should be full. A trainer with a dog on a short leash nears the shelter, where the assistant hides. At the signal, the assistant, holding a piece of meat in his left hand and a rod behind his back in his right hand, leaves the shelter and goes to the dog, calls its nickname, and offers her meat. If the dog tries to take food, the assistant stabs it with a blunt rod and leaves for cover. A few minutes later, he goes out again and offers the dog meat. If the dog tries to take food, the trainer gives the command "Stop!" and makes a jerk with the leash, and the assistant strikes with a rod and leaves. At this time, the trainer gives the command "Stop!"

This exercise is done daily, changing assistants. Approaching the dog, they try to diversify their actions (they approach calmly, run, or sneak). At the same time, they use different food. Also, change the location of the classes.

Then the dog develops the skill not to take food thrown by strangers. For this, food is not offered by hand. The assistant throws the food. Then they proceed according to the described method.

After practicing the exercises, conduct classes, throwing up food in the absence of a trainer, who ties the dog and hides. If a dog tries to take food thrown up in the absence of a trainer, he gives a sharp command "Stop!" and, if necessary, makes a strong jerk with a long leash attached to the collar.

The skill is considered developed if a dog without a leash in the presence of its trainer and without the trainer or owner refuses any food that is given by outsiders from their hands or thrown.

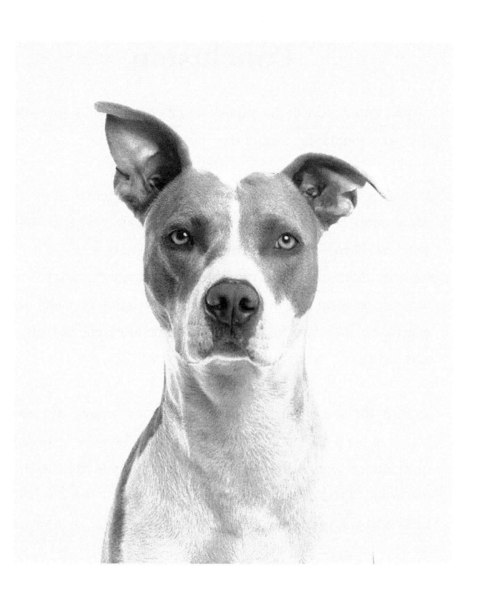

# Conclusion

As you know, a dog is an extension of its owner and I am certain that you would like to share the joy of such a contact.

It was my great love for dogs, my gratitude to them as companions, faithful companions, comrades in games, as well a servants, hard workers, and defenders who were ready to sacrifice themselves, that prompted me to write this book. In my opinion, an ideal dog should be, on the one hand, obedient, non aggressive, and cheerful, and on the other, alert, courageous, and physically strong.

In turn, the owner must be responsible for every step and every action of his pet. That is why the book gives the most important foundations, cementing the psychological unity of the dog and its owner. If you can do them religiously, you will achieve such unity and you will love your dog more.

In my opinion, a dog is more than just a pet. What is a man without dogs? If all the dogs disappeared, I believe a man would have died out from great loneliness of his spirit.

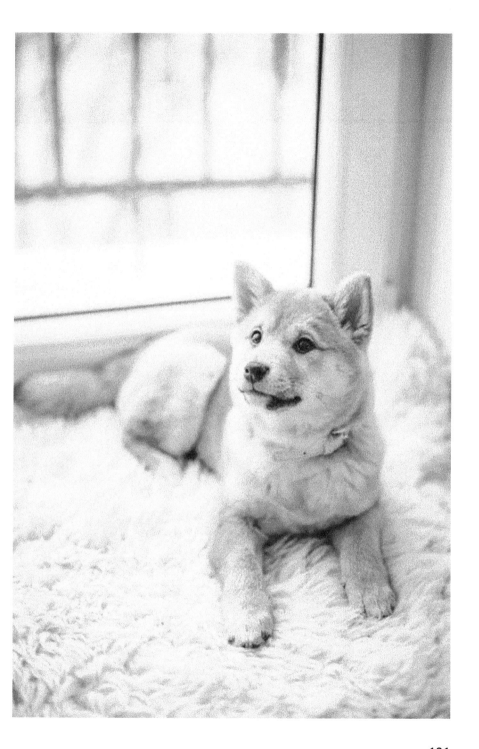

Lightning Source UK Ltd.
Milton Keynes UK
UKHW022049190121
377353UK00003B/320

9 781914 284557